Enough Already!

HOW TO LOSE WEIGHT ONCE
AND FOR ALL AND RECLAIM YOUR LIFE

ZALI NASH

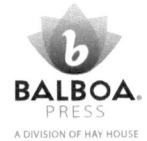

BALBOA
PRESS
A DIVISION OF HAY HOUSE

Balboa Press books may be ordered through booksellers or by contacting:

Balboa Press
A Division of Hay House
1663 Liberty Drive
Bloomington, IN 47403
www.balboapress.com.au
1-(877) 407-4847

ISBN: 978-1-4525-1122-1 (sc)
ISBN: 978-1-4525-1124-5 (hc)
ISBN: 978-1-4525-1123-8 (e)

Library of Congress Control Number: 2013915009

Printed in the United States of America

Balboa Press rev. date: 10/21/2013

To Jeremy, Charlie Chops,
Bushy, and Dad, for all your love

CONTENTS

INTRODUCTION

This book is for anyone who, like me, is fed up with constant dieting. I was frustrated and bemused seeing my friends, colleagues, students, and myself go on a diet, lose weight, and then put it all back on with a dollop of extra fat on the side for good measure. It doesn't matter if we are trying to lose three kilos or one hundred—studies from universities like UCLA have shown books and programs that just deal with diet and exercise will help us lose weight, but they won't keep the weight off long term. In fact, numerous studies suggest we will end up putting extra weight on. The catch is that until we address the issues behind the weight gain—I mean the real, meaty bones of the issues—we can try every program and read every book, but we will still find ourselves putting on the weight again and then some. If you have tried all the programs and diets under the sun and you are over it—I mean really over it—and if you are ready to reclaim your life and fill it with joy and happiness, then this is the book for you.

As a yoga teacher, I have with worked with scores of people struggling with their weight. I have witnessed and felt the pain, the frustration, the anger, and the blame that come when they keep sabotaging their own attempts to lose weight. What I am always really listening to is an insatiable hunger to come back to the true self, a desire to shed the kilos of pain that they may be hiding behind and to drop the layers of guilt over deeds gone wrong. For many, I am listening to an ache to strip off once and for all the drudgery of an unfulfilled life.

The inspiration for this book came from a beautiful young woman. Let's call her Sarah. I worked with Sarah for about eighteen months as her boss in my corporate life. She was immensely overweight. She was always on a different diet, slurping away at different green goos and chemical-laden chocolate shakes. She had pictures on her desk of a slimmer, glowing self who exuded confidence and joy. I could see the pain she was in, hidden behind a sassy, bold facade. We did lots of work on developing her professional skills at that time. She had motivation and ambition to burn. Yet she was moody, self-sabotaging, and, underneath it all, red, raw, and aching from the pain she was in. I eventually found out that she had been raped.

It all made sense to me. The layers of fat kept her safe from straying male eyes. The additional chunkiness was there for her to snuggle into, to comfort her, to keep the pain stuffed down deep inside. Her moodiness was her true self's tantrums at what she was doing to herself. She ached and hungered to become all that she could. I never took the chance to work this through with Sarah. It wasn't my role at the time. So this one's for you, Sarah.

This program has been exclusively developed to feed our true self's hunger for our own self-love.

It is a guide to identifying some of the root causes of overeating. It will give everyone the tools to make some behavioural changes to diet and exercise, not because you have to, but because part of you craves it. The dietary and exercise component will be almost effortless—like a by-product or secondary consideration. It is time to step into your potential and become all that you can. It is time to take life by the big, juicy lips and give it a big kiss hello.

The two ways to get the chunk off the body are without doubt (1) exercise and (2) food.

Yes, this book gets stuck into these two categories as well. We look at both of these sections from a new, empowering perspective.

The most important bits to me, the bits that will make the skin shimmer with happiness, are the bits that *keep* the weight off and, most importantly, hopefully bring us joy. These are

- dealing with any baggage and rot from the past,
- learning to accept, love, and like ourselves,
- living in the present moment every day, and
- beginning to live the life we are meant to.

To allow you to seamlessly experience the meditation, some exercises and yoga podcasts are available at www.pathtocontentment.com.

There is also a little terrier of a chapter at the end detailing what to do if you hit the wall. This is the chapter to read when you have had enough and want to cry and have a whole tub of ice cream—and it will tell you what to do just in case you do have that ice cream.

Summon up your strength and courage and a new attitude for success in this program. Here are the guidelines:

- Do not criticise, punish, or judge—ever.
- Forget about outcomes, and just go on the journey. See if you can just enjoy the time you are spending on this rather than concentrate on how much weight you have lost.
- If you happen to fall off the horse, jump back on. Every single breath is a new moment and an opportunity to start again. Each moment is a chance to take another step. In other words, just keep going.
- This program can be really challenging, because it not only deals with food and exercise, but also tackles the very reasons for weight

gain—and these things can be tough and grisly to deal with. You may also be changing conditioned patterns of behaviour that have been around for years. So, stay with it, jump on the website, and get lots of support. Join the forums. You are not alone. Many have gone before you, and many will come after you. Even though no one will have your exact journey, many can help along the way.

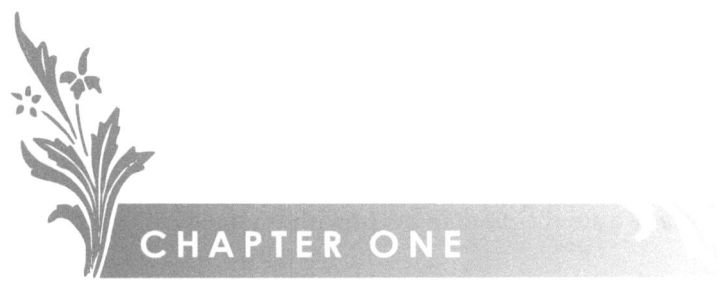

CHAPTER ONE

The Food Bit

On this program, we eat anything we want, with mindfulness and purpose. Yep, that's right—anything we want. If you want some chocolate, have some chocolate. In Deepak Chopra's book *Reinventing the Body, Resurrecting the Soul*, he says that as soon as we start to dictate to ourselves what we should and should not be eating, we can begin to set ourselves up for intense personal conflict, for there is a part of us that wants to live healthily and reach our potential. This is a part that wants to set up new healthy, empowering eating patterns in our brain. This immediately comes into conflict with well-worn neural pathways of conditioned eating that say, "When I am miserable, I reach for a double chocolate chip cookie with a gooey, runny centre." This is a pattern I may have had for years. Therefore, when I stop myself from eating like this, I am coming up against years of conditioned behaviour, and this causes all sorts of conflict and negative emotions. As soon as I start to deprive myself of anything, I want it more. With me it becomes an all-out obsession. I start to think about that chocolate bar *all* the time. I berate myself. I call myself every name in the swear bear jar. I have a dreadful day, rather than just getting on with it and being in the moment. The key to it all is, of course, portion size and the enjoyment of each and every mouthful of that treat. Try to cultivate mindfulness at all times. We want to step over all

1

that conflict and instead develop a practical, liveable way of eating forever that feeds the body and the heart without conflict. Then we will be able to examine, over time and with great awareness, why we want the triple pepperoni pizza. Then that pattern of behaviour will no longer be relevant, because the reason we ate the pizza to begin with is gone.

Delicious morsels of food aside, it is all about moving to whole, fresh, and, when possible and affordable, organic tucker.

If you are like any of my clients, you have tried every diet under our lovely sun, so you know all there is to know about food and nutrition. I have not gone into a lot of the whys in the food bit, because I presume you know it, and because the topic of sugar alone is enough to fill a whole book. However, if you would like further explanations for things, I do write a lot about food in my blog. There you will find studies, further reading suggestions and reasoning, and a lot more detailed information.

Here are the guidelines for eating:

- This program is all about eating whole foods. Give away to friends or to a shelter all the food items whose ingredients feature more numbers than foods you actually recognise. Fill the fridge to overflowing with veggies, lean meat and fish (preferably organic or free range), cheese, healthy bread (yes, the stuff with grains in it), free-range eggs, and organic milk. Fill the pantry with beans, lentils, spices, and organic flours. If you are vegetarian, terrific— the health benefits are tremendous. Just substitute your usual vegetable protein sources for selected organic grains, legumes, beans, dairy, and soy.
- Select a few things you *love* that you regard as treats. For the duration of the program, allow yourself to have one treat a day. The portion size is small.

- Eat more protein and fewer carbohydrates. That is, lean, organic meat, fish, nuts, seeds, legumes, whole-fat dairy (yes, whole fat—it is more filling and has extra vitamins we can't get in low-fat products, such as vitamin D), and eggs. Aim for a serving of one of these with each meal. A serving should be about the size of the palm of the hand.

- Limit your high-glycaemic carbohydrates (that is, the chippies, white flour pasta, white rice, pastries, and white bread) to just a few servings a week.

- Reduce your sugar intake. Try some lovely natural alternatives like stevia, molasses, maple syrup, and pear concentrate. You use heaps less and still get a delicious flavour.

- Incorporate some probiotic foods into your meals every day. Kefir, yoghurt, yoghurt drinks, aged cheese, cottage cheese, kimchi, and pickled vegetables are good options. They are so good for the immune system and also will help ease the bloat and make you, ah, "regular."

- Eat lots of prebiotic foods as well—otherwise, the probiotic foods don't work (raw garlic, onion, raw wheat bran, leeks, bananas, etc.).

- Incorporate stacks of fresh herbs into everything. I like to grow them in the kitchen so I can pluck them as I need them. A friend of mine has them growing amongst her flowers. Throw them in your salads, your casseroles—any chance you can add some in. Green herbs are wonderful for detoxifying the liver.

- Eat lots of spices. They are good sources of antioxidants. Turmeric is wonderful.

- Get yourself some natural fibre. Oat bran and wheat bran are great. Add it to smoothies, porridge, or yoghurt. It helps to keep you cleansed and on time in the bowel department again.

- Aim for two pieces of fruit a day. Half a cup of berries counts as one piece of fruit.

Go through the recipe books or jump on the www.pathtocontentment.com website, see what recipes others love, decide what you want to make, and go for it. I also love recipes by Jamie Oliver and Stephanie Alexander for their whole-food approaches to eating. They are passionate about eating whole foods and also give great instructions on growing your own veggies and fruit. There is no special list of meals to eat on certain days in a unique magical order. You know what to do. You know what you like and what your family will eat. If you find a recipe you love, send it in so we can put it on the website. Photos are great too.

There are so many things you can make. If you feel like a lasagne, then make lasagne. But instead of having the usual serving, have a little slice with a *huge* salad and maybe an egg, or doctor the recipe to be really healthy. Never deny yourself food. Just stick to the principles, and all will be tops.

- Eat **h**eaps of veggies.
- **E**at a good dose of protein at every meal.
- **A**dd a tablespoon of oat bran or wheat bran to a meal every day.
- **L**imit all refined, highly processed foods, white breads, pasta, rice, and sugar.
- Eat **t**wo pieces of fruit a day.
- **H**ave at least a litre and a half of water a day.

Make your shopping list and just forget about the food. This is really important. Instead of spending time thinking about meals, calories, and portion sizes, just enjoy the process of preparation. There is nothing in that cupboard or fridge that will harm you. The whole idea is to stick to the principles and then let go of the deprivation and the worry and the measuring portions and the *bluh*. Enjoy food.

I used to be a low-carb convert. I avoided all carbs of any sort, and it worked for me. It worked really well. I shed kilos and toned up a treat.

Then I noticed that my bowels weren't working regularly. I kept getting sick all the time, and my skin wasn't the best, despite the water, the lotions and potions, and the fish oil.

I then went to a naturopath who convinced me to start eating a lot more grains and beans and pulses. She also talked me into to having two pieces of fruit a day and adding in the probiotics and prebiotics. I was quite frankly very doubtful! I thought those kilos would start piling on. But to my surprise and delight, not only did I lose weight, but my health also took a leapfrog bound. People were telling me how good I looked. More importantly, I felt good. So get into that fruit, those lentils, and those chickpeas. You will be surprised!

Just like we clean our homes, our bodies need a deep clean too. Our bodies encounter hundreds of chemicals, toxins, and bacteria every day. These make their way into our body through our skin (just think how nicotine patches work), our food and drink, and the air we breathe. All these unwanted things hang around in there as waste. The longer the waste and toxins linger, the longer they slowly leech all that rot into our system. This affects our immune system, our endocrine system, our organs, our skin, our nervous system, and even our reproductive system with all the synthetic hormones we consume.

With our butts lovingly lounging in chairs most of the day and us not eating very much fibre and drinking more coffee than water, all that unexpelled rot and those toxins tend to hang around in the lower intestines, coat the organs, and make life a rather gassy, bloated affair. All this impedes our bodies' ability to work at their best. The chemicals and waste build up, which can make our bodies find it harder to assimilate nutrients, and our immune systems can also suffer as result. We may get sicker more often. We may find it more difficult to cope with the major stressors of life. These are not the right conditions for us to slip into our authentic selves.

We know when we feel sluggish. Our tummies are so bloated we are uncomfortable and the skin under our eyes is like two saggy, yellow or blue-black pillows. When I get a brain fog and constant colds and look about four months pregnant, I know it is time for some intestinal cleaning—nothing radical like a juice fast, but a gentle, pure vegetable intake just for a day. It is a wonderful way to begin again and to honour my body.

Pick a day, preferably one when you aren't working or caring for little people by yourself. It needs to be when you haven't got too much on. (Weekends are always good.) On this day eat nothing but energy and vitamin-packed veggies from start to finish. This day should ideally feel like a retreat day. This is difficult, I know, particularly if you have a family. There are some suggestions for it in the guidelines.

Beforehand, though, a release-and-surrender day is a good time to say goodbye, not only to the physical contaminants in our systems, but also to the things we wish out of our lives. The exercise below will to help you do this.

The Surrender Ceremony (before the Detox Day)

What You'll Need

- a journal (Any blank notepad will do, but one with a lovely cover would make it that much more special.)
- short strips of paper
- a pen
- a flameproof bowl
- music
- a lighter or matches

What Next?

List on small pieces of paper what you think are your triggers for overeating. What or who makes you reach for a double chocolate chip cookie without even thinking? Take note of any situations when you like to wrap yourself in cosiness and chow down on something delicious. What habits do you have that involve eating? Write down any emotions and words that you are stuffing down with food. Add to that anything else that you want to change or get rid of about yourself (nothing physical here)—things you would like to change about how you act and react in times of negativity. Consider also how you respond in circumstances that are out of your control. Write down as many things as you can think of that are holding you back or that you would like to let go of in your life.

Think about

- behaviours,
- eating patterns,
- work routines,
- negative self-talk,
- feelings like jealousy, revenge, and spite, and
- the issues that you talk to yourself negatively about.

Prioritise these from the trivial to the dinosaur stuff.

List all of these things on individual strips of paper. Then, with great reverence, pick up each slip of paper. Read it and allow the emotional response to come with it. Be with that emotion. Allow yourself to feel it. Then take a deep breath and place each piece of paper into a flameproof bowl, saying to yourself, "I release myself from [insert what is on the slip of paper]." Shut your eyes and visualise each of these things rising up in smoke and disappearing. See your heart opening and a smile coming to rest upon your face. Next, take a lighter and set fire to the pile. As the smoke rises up, visualise all those unhealthy patterns and feelings disappearing. Thank those old habits and feelings for the lessons they have taught you. Then imagine that their departure has created a wonderful space in the deepest part of you—a space that your potential and growth will now step into. The fire would by now have burnt out, so place the ashes onto a potted plant or into your garden to be returned to the earth and recycled into something new and nourishing.

The Day of Surrender and Release

What You'll Need

- heaps and heaps of bright, gorgeous veggies and salad (Find a market and buy locally or organically if you can afford it. No potatoes, corn, or pumpkin. You want lots of greens, oranges, reds, and purples. Include garlic, chilli (if you like it), carrots, celery, spinach, and Asian greens.)
- a juicer (If you don't have one, borrow one for the day, or find a local juice shop and get them to do the juice for you.)
- all-natural veggie stock and spices
- a lemon
- lots of fresh herbs
- herbal teas (not fruit teas or chai) (Think peppermint, chamomile, mint (mint leaves in hot water is a truly delicious drink), crushed cardamom pods, and rosehips.)
- your favourite music
- essential oils that smell right for you (I love lavender, orange, rose geranium, and patchouli.)
- a scented candle that smells good
- a cloth serviette

- a vase and a flower
- a body scrub and a lovely thick body moisturiser
- a nice plate, bowl, glass, and set of cutlery
- your journal and pen

What Next?

- Begin the day with a meditation. Simply find a quiet spot away from distractions and a position that is comfortable for you and breathe deeply for five minutes. Allow your mind to focus on your breath. Whenever a thought comes in, let it come in and then let it go.
- Put music on—something soothing and calming.
- Burn some essential oils—anything that smells right.
- When it's time to shower or bathe, use a body scrub in strong upward strokes towards the heart and gentle circling motion around the chest.
- Lather moisturising cream on your body, paying special attention to the tootsies and hands.
- Throughout the day drink lots of water and herbal tea. Avoid coffee, green tea, and black tea.
- Every time some sort of food or beverage crosses those lips during this day, give thanks. Every droplet and morsel is to be honoured, treasured, and celebrated. Nothing is taken for granted.
- Set yourself a place at the table. Use a cloth serviette and put a flower and a candle on the table. Play music. Drink water out of a wine glass. Eat each meal here. If you live with others, then set the table for them too!
- Make yourself a cup of soothing warm water and lemon. Sit down when you drink it. Feel the steam against your cheeks. Allow every mouthful to be savoured.

- Before you prepare a meal, snack, or drink, place all the ingredients on the table and look at the colours and textures. If you have fresh herbs, smell them. Think about where the food has come from. What has gone into bringing it to you? What a privilege it is to have these wonderful foods before you. One breakfast idea is some mushrooms and spinach lightly sautéed with garlic and fresh thyme served with a tomato, avocado, and basil salsa.
- In the morning go for a nice, slow walk or do some gentle, restorative yoga. There is a program for you on the website.
- For a midmorning snack, have carrot, celery, and beetroot juice and some vegetable sticks to munch on.
- For lunch, if it is hot, then eat a lovely, large salad with lots of herbs and colour. If it is cold, have a pot of heart-warming soup.

Vegetable Soup Recipe

What You'll Need

- lots of vegetables
- garlic
- water
- spices and herbs

What Next?

Lightly sauté any garlic or onion. Then chop up your veggies, pop them in the pot, add your herbs and spices to taste, and bring everything to a boil. Reduce the heat and simmer for twenty minutes to an hour. Then get your handheld food processor out, turn the heat off, and blend until it comes to a nice, thick, smooth consistency.

- Fill the afternoon with gentle activities. Read some of your favourite books or magazines. Have long baths. Lie in the garden or head to the beach. Just take it easy.
- For afternoon tea, have a nice juice. This time, try celery, carrot, spinach, and tomato with some pepper. Munch on some vegetable sticks.
- For dinner, steam a large plate of vegetables or do a stir-fry.

Stir-Fry Recipe

What You'll Need

- a tablespoon of grated ginger
- one clove of crushed garlic
- chilli (optional)
- any vegetables (Good ones are mushrooms, finely sliced carrot, bok choy or any Asian greens, snow peas, beans, and bean sprouts.)
- coriander (optional)

What Next?

Lightly fry the garlic, ginger, and chilli. Add in the rest of the vegetables and cook briskly on high, turning them constantly until just tender. Add in your chopped coriander and stir through. Yum!

- After dinner, make yourself a soothing cup of chamomile tea. Burn some lavender oil. Lights some candles around the house. Put on some soothing background music.
- Meditate in the evening. Take yourself off to where you did your morning meditation and light a candle. Remind yourself of what you are releasing and just follow your breath for ten minutes.

- Before bed, do some journaling. How are you feeling? What did you enjoy about today? What did you struggle with? What did you surrender and release? Did you find yourself obsessing over some food or having battles with yourself? Did you have any other thoughts and revelations? One of my clients, Sarah, found this day extremely emotional and found herself wanting to cry a lot. This is normal. Let it all out, and if you feel like having a gut-wrenching sob, go for it. Try some journaling along with it to see if you can articulate the cause of the emotion. It doesn't matter if you can't. It is just good to get the emotion felt, acknowledged, and released.
- Snuggle into bed.

If you have little people or big, long, hungry people (in the form of teenagers) to take care of, then do what you can. Maybe watch a movie and read lots of books with the kids. Do some crafts and get them to help make some wild and wacky juice creations with you. If you have little people who snooze, then why not snooze too? Head out to a park and lie in the grass as they charge around. Go for a slow, long walk. With big people it is much easier. Maybe they can arrange their own transport to and from things for the day and bring you a nice cup of herbal tea and a kiss—well, OK, maybe a grunt.

Please note that it is normal as our bodies cleanse themselves to feel a little light-headed, weak, and tired. I quite often get a headache. This is our bodies getting rid of the rot. Rest.

There is one more point, and it is a big one. When I did this the first time, the things that were the hardest to deal with were my attitudes towards deprivation that I talked about earlier. All those feelings and struggles I used to have when I dieted came to the surface. The day was spent obsessing over food, resenting what I was eating, and looking for any excuse to eat something else and do something else. I was horrified with how obsessed and grumpy I was about doing the cleanse. It was quite simply dreadful.

Throughout the day, pay lots of attention to what is coming up. Observe the inner monologue that occurs when you devote yourself to a day of veggies. This is just some of what goes through our mind when we diet! Try not to judge yourself if this happens. Instead, listen with compassion and love and start to ask yourself why you feel like this.

One of the best ways to overcome this is to change the paradigm and think of it as a pampering day rather than a detox day. It really is all about motivation, attitude, and intention. That is why the meditation, the surrender ceremony beforehand, and the loving, pampering care are so important. When we look at these twenty-four hours as a day of self-love and care and a chance to nourish, cleanse, and renew, there is no place for the old self-sabotaging behaviours to sink their pearly whites in. Every time the self-destructive thoughts start to come in, observe them neutrally and with love and compassion and then bring yourself back to the intention and to what is being let go.

Food and Guilt

Guilt and food like to pair up from time to time. There may be moments when we slip into ways of eating that are driven by something other than hunger. This sometimes occurs consciously, sometimes not. The worst bit, though, is that after a whole double cheese and salami pizza has been stuffed in the gut, the guilt washes in. Everyone has different outward responses to guilt. Some people get defensive and aggressive at the world. Others berate themselves, beating up on what is left of their self-esteem, whilst some withdraw a little more into the land of numbness.

Guilt and food really have no reason to be together at any time. It is a waste of energy and precious minutes. For example, say you had some double chocolate chip muffins with fresh cream and vanilla ice cream. Big whoop. Just breathe in again and remember that the next moment is new. Life is not meant to categorised or sorted into good and bad, pure and dirty, healthy and unhealthy. It is simply life. The muffin, just like life, is neither good nor bad. It is just a muffin. Whatever the reasons for eating the muffin, let's allow ourselves the freedom to live without guilt over what food we eat. We have not done a *bad* thing. We just ate a muffin—maybe even twenty muffins. The key is that we make sure we enjoy them, treasure them, relish them. If you are aware that you are eating the muffin, you might want to ask yourself why. Do this in a curious, non-judgemental way. If no answer is forthcoming, let it go. Don't take those moments of chocolate loveliness for granted, and move on. The next breath taken is a new moment where we get to consciously choose all over again how we will live.

I Treat Myself

What You'll Need:

- a few favourite treats that you love to eat

What Next?

- Every day allow yourself a small portion of your favourite treat. Pick the same time each day, and allow yourself to be fully focussed on eating the treat. Think about who made the treat and the resources, time, and care that went to getting it into your hands. Look at this morsel of delectable culinary delight. When you hold it in your hands or mouth, what does it feel like? Then

14

place it in your mouth and just allow yourself to taste it without chewing. Then start chewing and notice the texture of the food as you chomp and the rhythm of your jaw. What does your tongue do? What flavours can you taste? How does this make you feel? What thoughts flow through your mind while you are enjoying this little bit of deliciousness?

Repeat this exercise every time you decide to have your treat.

Succulent and Sacred Eating

What You'll Need

- your nose
- music
- your mouth, taste buds
- your hands
- your ears
- your eyes
- time
- gratitude

What Next?

Every time you eat from here on out, it is to be a whirligig for the senses, just as you do now with your daily treat. This starts right at the beginning with food preparation. Feel the ingredients. Smell some of them. Take a bite of the fresh veggies or fruit. Savour the bite. Listen to the crunch as your teeth sink into the flesh of the food. Enjoy the sound as the knife chops. Let your eyes soak up the colours.

As you cut, chop, slice, stir, and sniff, watch the colours and feel the heat of the stove. As you create your culinary masterpiece, feel the weight of the implements in your hand.

Say a blessing as you prepare the meal for all those who will eat it and all those who have contributed to the preparation.

Then, decorate the table and make it beautiful with flowers, placemats, a tablecloth, or a runner. Use your nice plates and bowls and crockery.

If it is possible, wait until everyone is present and eat, taste, slurp, savour, mull, and chew together. Every bite is to be feasted on and dedicated to your body and well-being with awareness. Taste the combinations of flavours, chew your food until it has almost melted away, and swallow with deliberateness.

Feel your eating implements in your hands. Place them down between mouthfuls. Be present with those you are eating with.

Bring your awareness to your belly and know when you are sated.

What happens if everything isn't eaten? Well, there are lots of productive options. Pets, compost, and leftovers are just a few. There is no need to feel guilt for leaving something on your plate.

A Sacred Space

The kitchen is one of the most heart-centred rooms in a house. It is a place where family often gathers to chat while food is prepared and, depending on the size of the kitchen, even eaten. I often have people draped over benches chatting away or having a cup of tea and a chat while I prepare food. The preparation of tucker is not just about making meals, but about preparing dishes that nourish the body and the heart as well.

Given the importance of food to our lives, the kitchen is a great spot to set up a little sacred space—a place that reminds us visually of the commitment to this new way of eating and living. Every time we walk into the kitchen we will be reminded of who we are and what is important to us in terms of eating and nourishing ourselves and those we love.

What You'll Need

- a nice bowl, dish, or jar
- a vase
- beautiful blossoms
- a selection of fresh, in-season produce or just-baked healthy treats
- a photo of someone you love with you in it
- some potted herbs (optional)
- inspirational quotes

What Next?

Find a lovely, light-filled space in the kitchen. Place the bowl and vase there along with the picture. Fill the vase and bowl with flowers and some juicy, in-season fruit or some of your own healthy baking. Place any of your quotes here as well. Make it look beautiful and inspiring. This is the in-kitchen reminder of all you are becoming. It visually prompts you to eat well. It taps you on the shoulder and says you are becoming your potential. It is the soft whisper of remembrance that every mouthful nourishes and sustains you—that every bite is a choice. It will serve as a place of inspiration and dedication every time you enter the kitchen. It is a place where you can marvel at the colours, textures, and smells of food and bring gratitude into the preparation of your dishes.

Making Your Own Treats

What You'll Need

- some creativity
- time
- a recipe and all the stuff for your favourite treats
- music

What Next?

There is something so much more special about home-baked or—prepared goodies. I think maybe it is the time and effort that go into the preparation. The title of this exercise is self-explanatory, really. So whether your foody treasure is sweet or savoury, get busy. If you already make your own treat, go through the recipe and substitute what you can for healthier ingredients. For instance, if your treat is something baked, try replacing white sugar with a healthier alternative. Replace conventional flour with organic and then maybe over time change to a different type of flour. Experiment and have fun. What is wonderful about this is that you know exactly what is going into the treat. You know it contains no chemicals or additives. You may also appreciate it a lot more when you eat it, as you know the effort and time it took to make it. Don't forget to make some for family and friends and send your favourite healthy treat recipe in to me to pop on the website.

Become a Whole-Food Lover

As the true self takes the driver's seat, the way we prefer to eat may change. It may evolve as we tune into what our bodies want and don't want. Junk food was my soul's balm for a long time. After a hard day I would reach for anything deep-fried and salty and then follow it with the smooth, cool deliciousness of ice cream. Now, I trundle off for some meditation and a cup of herbal tea.

This way of life is about us eating what we want to—having our treats, continuing our internal work, sating the hunger in us with what we really crave emotionally, and getting rid of the labels and just enjoying life. It is about releasing ourselves from any guilt and fear as all the reasons for overeating become slowly irrelevant. You'll reach a point in your life where you no longer want to put things into your body that aren't good for it. This happened with me very gradually. I might have been halfway through a Snickers bar when I decided I didn't want any more. I couldn't really taste it. It was no longer the peanuty, caramel moment of bliss that that first bite was. I realised as I automatically padded out to the freezer on my nightly ice cream vigil that I wasn't really hungry. If you are anything like me, this will happen mouthful by mouthful, without any thoughts of deprivation. In fact, it may not involve much thought at all. Your body knows how to reach its best weight and what it needs to be healthy!

Daily Checklist

The Food Bit

- Eat **h**eaps of veggies.
- **E**at a good dose of protein at every meal.
- **A**dd a tablespoon of oat bran or wheat bran to a meal every day.
- **L**imit all refined, highly processed foods, white breads, pasta, rice, and sugar.
- Eat **t**wo pieces of fruit a day.
- **H**ave at least a litre and a half of water a day.

- Don't forget the treat every day, and if you can, make it. Fall in love with fresh, delicious whole food again.
- Enjoy mindful sensory eating. Make every plate of deliciousness a dining pleasure for your senses.

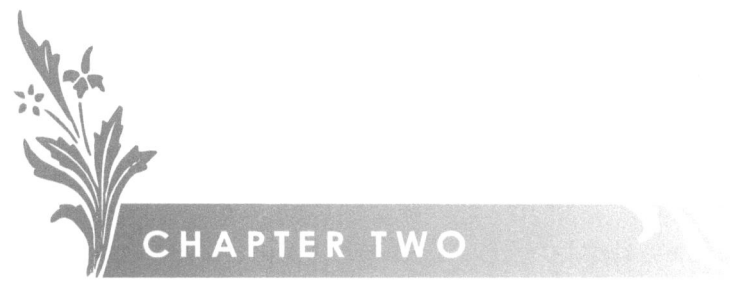

CHAPTER TWO

The Dealing-with-Past-Baggage-and-Rot Bit

In the heart-centred approach to weight loss, we really focus on utilising our potential. To be able to do that, we have to start to love ourselves, to believe we deserve all the great things that utilising our talents and attributes brings us.

A big part of this is self-acceptance. In this section you will begin to break out of the shackles of past hurts and pain. These cause all sorts of emotional roadblocks like fear, resentment, anger, sadness, and jealousy—roadblocks we often use food to detour around.

Most of these shackles can be dealt with via two strategies:

1. Forgiveness
2. Letting go of what doesn't serve us. That means surrendering the past hurts that we often lug around as emotional baggage.

In this part, we will also open our hearts up to any feelings of fear that we may be experiencing. We will learn how to work with fear and use it is as a catalyst to reclaim our lives and step into all that we can be.

That means really gnawing at the bones of our issues and tackling stuff at a deeper lever as well as at an everyday level.

We will set ourselves free of those feelings of pain, boredom, numbness, and fear when we let go of the reasons they came about to begin with. It is all about the surrender and release. First we need to surrender—we must acknowledge that it is time to move on. Then comes the release—we must set free all those experiences that have led to fears, boredom, and numbness. This will be done physically and spiritually. It can be as rapid or as slow and nurturing as needed. Our hearts and bodies will be our guide on this one, not our schedules or our egos.

This part of the program is a toughie but thoroughly rewarding and wonderfully empowering, perhaps even transforming. But it can be bloody hard. There, I have said it. So again, please treat yourself with love and gentleness during this bit. If you uncover things that are just too much, please seek a professional counsellor or therapist to help you work through it. What this section will do is help you on the journey to why you may be living as you are—why you haven't yet realised those dreams and stepped into that beautiful self deep within and taken claim of all that you can be.

Resentment and Guilt

Resentment and guilt are two of the most powerful negative emotions and are common reasons for eating too many slices of pepperoni pizza with double cheese. In my case they used to work together, playing tag team on my spirit until I had no energy left, little love left in the tank, and no self-esteem to speak of—just a dribble of self, reaching for something that will make me feel better. Resentment and guilt like to play like a song on repeat every day too, reminding us at every opportunity how bad we should feel.

Guilt pops up in all sorts of situations, from the big—the greatest mistakes of our lives—to the smaller but no less significant, regarding exercise or better eating. Guilt is just a waste of time and energy. There is no point wallowing in the past. We cannot change it. Whatever happened has happened. We cannot physically go back and rectify the situation. So there really is no point in us wasting all those minutes, hours, and precious sleep moments thinking about how things could have been. It is just a drain on life. Instead, we should let go and focus on the lessons we can learn from the situation. I know—much easier said than done. But it's doable with practice (in my case, many years of practice). Every time I keep thinking about something that I regret or feel guilty about, I simply remind myself of the lesson I will take on board, take a deep breath, and continue on until the next time it pops up into my thoughts.

Being unable to forgive and resenting someone or our lives, however, is crueller to ourselves in some ways. When we harbour resentment and find it difficult to forgive, we really consume ourselves with negative emotions until our spirit hungers for release and comfort. Look, I know that letting go of pain and forgiving someone is one of the hardest things. These two emotions have little hooks that sink a little deeper into our tissues at every opportunity. I had one client whose husband cheated on her. The couple went to counselling initiated by the husband and worked really hard at reconciling. The counselling was working really well, but the client still harboured such pain and resentment towards her husband that she couldn't really move on in the relationship. It was only by allowing herself to grieve for what was lost, to vent and feel the emotions, that she was able to begin to forgive. Now they have a relationship that is stronger than before, and she is a lot more content with her life and who she is. All the counselling in the world won't help until we allow ourselves to feel and release that pain and move on. It's a very personal thing. This can take many months, even years. So how do we cope with this supressed pain, guilt, and resentment in the meantime? We shovel food in, compulsively shop for things we don't need, and surround ourselves with stuff.

Guilt-Catching Exercise

This exercise helps us to identify what role, if any, supressed pain, guilt, or resentment plays in our day-to-day lives.

What You'll Need

- a journal
- a pen

What Next?

Use your journal or a piece of paper if you are out and about. Every time you crave something you really do not want to eat, you skip your planned workout, or you do something that makes you feel guilty, take a note of the thought or action immediately before it. Also, when you begin to bury yourself in work, when you turn the telly on, when you decide to buy something you don't need—tune in to what happened just before it. You will know when to tune in, because you may feel the faintest whisper of disappointment, apathy, or regret deep inside. You may also feel a sledgehammer in your tummy, depending on the extent of the numbing activity.

For many people, the reasons for overeating are guilt, resentment, and an inability to release pain from past experiences. Becoming aware that this is even happening is the first step in letting go of this pain. The next step is allowing yourself to feel the pain, and to do that you should aim to overcome the fear behind the pain. The fear of feeling the pain is often much more powerful in stopping you from moving forward than the experience of the pain itself. The reason for this is that you are not the person you were when the painful experience first happened, but your fear may react as though you are. For many who may not have had the happiest of childhoods, it is in fact the three-year-old self who still fears the same experience happening or the feeling the pain again. That three-year-old self is mighty different from who you are now. Even the self who was devastated by a broken relationship a few months ago is very different from who you are now. Just the process of noting your trigger will assist you in becoming aware of any issues associated with overeating or self-sabotage.

How to Cope with the Fears That Prevent Us from Forgiving and Moving On

What You'll Need

- courage
- a journal
- a pen

What Next?

In your journal, explore the following.

- Take a moment to think about the experience you are trying to let go of or the person you are trying to forgive, if forgiveness and resentment are an issue. Allow yourself to feel any fear when you do. Gently conduct a mental scan of your body and notice how it is feeling. Is there tightness anywhere? Has the fear settled somewhere physically? Do you feel nauseated or acidic in the tummy? What is your heart rate doing? Then take it further, by asking yourself the following questions:

- What is the ultimate root cause of the fear?
- What would happen if this fear came true?
- What can you do to cope with the overwhelming feeling of fear if it arises?
- How can you physically ease the symptoms of the fear? Use point one above to help identify physical places the fear has settled in.
- What can you do to address this fear and allow yourself to move on to forgiveness and letting go of that pain?

To give you some inspiration, here is what I use to process negative emotions and fears when they arise. Negative emotions and fears in my own life usually pop up when I least expect it and bite me on the bum.

For example, let's just say hypothetically I was finding it really hard to forgive someone in my family for constant psychological abuse. I begin to think about the experience and the person and allow the fear to be felt. That fear is that of a young girl about ten years old, a girl who desperately doesn't want to relive that pain. When I feel like this, my throat gets very tight. I clench my jaw and I grit my teeth. I also feel a sensation of jitteriness that is almost panic-like in my gut. I get all agitated. I identified this by noticing how when someone puts me down, I often reach for something to soothe me, like a cookie. I replay the conversation over and over. I put myself down and make jokes about myself so that I can denigrate myself rather than someone else. I ignore the compliments people give me. I don't even ignore them—I incinerate them before they have a chance even to enter the atmosphere. The root cause of this fear may be that when I was a child I was berated and uncared for by an abusive parent and never felt worthy. To address the situation, I start to become aware of how often I paint a negative picture of myself, using my journal and through my daily meditation.

I do a body scan and see where it is in my physical body I am holding tension or if there is an ache or a pain anywhere. I either relax the muscles or meditate on it, using my breath and visualisation skills to send a shining light or a sense of expansiveness into the area to create some space and ease the tension.

I then comfort myself when this happens and ask myself whether this fear is really relevant now. I soothe and talk gently to myself, letting myself express the pain and fear. Then I write all that down in my journal. I encourage myself and do something physical to release the emotion. It may be anything from shaking my hands vigorously to doing some yoga poses. The other day I was feeling extremely agitated and anxious about something and did ten rounds of sun salute (a common yoga sequence) to help physically express and process the anxiety. I used that anxiety as fuel to power me through the sequence.

I then go and do something nice for myself. This is really important. It may be making myself a cup of tea, treating myself to a bath, or just listening to music for a few minutes.

What I would then do is start to actively concentrate on my good points instead of my fear of being unlovable. I would consciously begin to claim acknowledgement and praise for work that I would previously have ignored or blocked. Instead of repeating to myself, "I am not very good at my job—she is just saying that," I would now repeat the compliment that the person said to me instead. Every time that fear pops up, I would create a vision about what could be achieved and what life would be like without this fear. That is where determination and motivation come from. Then I focus on the emotions that come with that vision.

I do this all the time now. It really helped me in my relationship with my husband, whom I had some self-sabotaging behaviour with. It has helped me really get rid of some limiting ideas I had about his perception of me and, more importantly, my perception of myself in our relationship.

This is a good exercise to come back to as you continue with the program or anytime you feel fear or anxiety arise in your life.

Here it is in instruction format:

- Allow yourself to feel the emotion.
- Comfort and console yourself.
- Feel where and how it is manifesting itself in your body. Breathe deeply into that and imagine sending a healing light into that area.
- Write about how you are feeling, talk to someone about it who will just listen, sing about it if you are musical, or draw it if you are artistic. Somehow express how you are feeling. Get it all out. Also express any past stuff that comes up with it as well. Get it all out.
- Comfort that hurt part of yourself, often there's a deep longing to be listened to and nurtured.
- Do something physical to release it from your body, such as deep breathing, shaking your hands, running, or doing yoga—anything your gut or your inner wisdom advises you to do.
- Then reward yourself with something wonderful. This is really important. It could be a bath, a massage, or a guided meditation. Buy yourself some flowers. Do something that nourishes you.
- Every time the fear comes up or you find yourself doing something self-sabotaging, create a vision of what it would be like without this fear, and concentrate on that.
- Allow yourself to do this as often as you need to, 'cause fear is a pain in the rump. It can keep coming up again and again, but it will fade with time, and eventually you can overcome it.

Righto, Fear Dealt With. So How Do I Forgive?

The steps so far have been acknowledging that there is something to let go and deciding to step into the fear and feel any suppressed pain. Then deal with any emotion and pain underneath and comfort and soothe yourself.

It is not just our fears that we stuff down with food. Often our hurt is hidden behind resentment and an inability to forgive. This can be tough stuff to deal with. It stains our souls, drains our spirits, and fuels our fat cells. The more we hold onto that pain manifesting as resentment and anger, the longer we hold onto our fat.

One of the greatest realisations in my life and in the lives of so many of my clients is that the only person who suffers from resentment and lack of forgiveness is the person experiencing it. Now is the time to free ourselves from that terrible act or that person. When we let go of these feelings, we are by no means condoning what was done to us, but we are finally freeing ourselves from what has occurred. We are the only ones holding us back with pain, anger, resentment, and hurt.

The first step in letting go is acknowledging the wisdom we have gained from the situation. How has it shaped us? Perhaps it has shaped our personality in a negative manner. Perhaps we have put up barriers for people to clamber over, booby traps for unsuspecting friends to fall into. When they do, we need to acknowledge that too and make some decisions about letting that go if it is holding us back. Then it's time to let go and make the ultimate decision to step out of the binds of hurt and into our potential. This one step will set you free.

Bye-Bye Guilt and Resentment

What You'll Need

- a pen
- a journal

What Next?

- Begin by jotting down any resentment you feel towards someone.
- Spend three or four minutes writing about how you feel. Just vomit it all out. Give it voice and expression, or draw it if it feels better to draw it. Don't censor it. Allow it to be bitter, vile, and dark.
- Now take a few breaths and just sit in silence, allowing the feelings to flow through you and also yourself to feel them.
- Feel where they settle in your body and how your body processes those feelings, just as we did in the releasing fear exercise.
- Consciously let them go through muscle release or the light visualisation exercise in the previous exercise.
- Do something physical to process the emotion. It could be deep breathing, jumping around, singing to loud music, punching a pillow, or running your guts out—whatever.
- Then offer yourself some comfort. Write to yourself about how sorry you are about the pain you're feeling or that you keep beating yourself up over something you cannot change.
- Write down all that you have learnt—the deeper wisdom. Not the "I am never going to trust that person again" or the "I am just an unworthy idiot who doesn't deserve friends" sorts of thoughts. That is the pain talking. What deep lessons have you learnt?
- Now give thanks for those lessons. You are a different person because of them.

- If it is self-forgiveness you need, then decide to honour the lessons you have learnt by moving forward and letting go of the remorse and self-abuse. These emotions will not change the past, but living as your best self will certainly ensure that you take on the lessons that can be gained from those emotions. If it is resentment, then make a decision that this person can no longer hurt you.

- It is time to start putting your energy into what you value rather than bitterness about things you cannot change. Create some boundaries in your life so that that person cannot hurt you anymore, and set yourself free.

In some cases, the pain and trauma of the past really should be processed with the help of a professional. They can be just so helpful in guiding you through this. This is tough stuff, and I wish you the very best for this part of the journey. Know that you are not alone, and feel free to share with others in our forum—or perhaps even encourage others who may be struggling with this section.

We create a lot of our baggage. The self-limiting baggage not only gives us reason to shovel the chips in, but it also significantly hinders us from reaching our true potential and being all that we can. That baggage is generally created by the thoughts that we like to replay over and over again. Like a track on repeat, we use it to justify our hurt, wrongs, and behaviour. The mind is such a powerful thing. A single thought can alter the chemistry in our bodies and the neural pathways in our brain and cause a change in our emotional state, health, and well-being. The following exercise is an example of the persuasiveness and control our thoughts can have if we let them.

The Power of Our Thoughts

What You'll Need

- imagination

What Next?

Think about brushing your teeth. Imagine picking up the toothbrush and squeezing the toothpaste on. Then see yourself brushing the bottom of the top teeth, behind the top teeth, the top of the bottom teeth, and behind the top teeth. Imagine brushing the fronts of the teeth. Have you noticed an excess of saliva sloshing around in your mouth? Has the need to spit or swallow suddenly become apparent? That is what I am talking about! You simply thought about brushing your teeth and your body responded accordingly. Imagine how our bodies respond when we think about how fat we are or how much we hate our bum! Every single thought about our bodies and relationships has physical and emotional implications for us! Our thoughts can reprogram our very cells, our patterns of behaviour, and how we treat people.

The ego likes to be correct about all things. Bless its cotton socks. It utilises our thoughts to support its claims about how right it is. The mind is really just a thought processor, churning out hundreds of thousands of bytes of information for us to believe or not—for us to regard or not. The choice is ours. Our lives are made up of hundreds of these beliefs based on thoughts, perceptions, and comments that we have agreed with, repeated, reinforced, and absorbed into our fat cells to make this truth become real.

Take this a step further. Let's say I was abused sexually, physically, or emotionally. This abuse could lead to a thought that I am not loved or valued. This thought could then repeat itself over and over in different ways as I seek justification for the abuse, often backed up by conversations I have with a friends who say something rude. Then there could follow an offhand remark from someone I work with. Pretty soon, I'd think to myself, *Well, hell, I really am unlovable.* So I'd stuff food in to soak up the pain or to gag the outrage at not feeling loved and to prevent it from erupting. I'd fill my mouth with all things delicious because I need to comfort and salve my suffering. The only way I can shelter from this abuse, from this perception of being unlovable that I have created, is to chow down on some cake. I believe subconsciously that cake is safe. Cake is good. Cake is love. But cake is not love. Cake is good, though—but cake is just cake. It's delicious, yes, but it is not love. It won't take away what we all truly hunger for: love.

Thought Catching

This is something that we will do throughout the whole program and will eventually become automatic.

What You'll Need

- a journal
- a pen
- lots of honesty

What Next?

From here on in, whenever you are splodging around in a splat of negativity or acting in a manner you didn't want to, or if you find yourself midmunch with a handful of deep-fried goodness you didn't even realise you had, observe what came before it. What triggered the reaction? Take a quick note of it in your journal. This could well be one of your roadblocks; this could well be one of your wounds. If you are having trouble working out what you ache for, this is a great way to find out.

- Observe your negative reaction to something.
- What the heck triggered that?
- Why do you feel that this is important? Why has it hurt?
- Label the wound.

Each week, review your journal, and over time you will find some patterns emerging. It is a great way to become aware of patterns that don't align with your true self and that you want to change. It is also vital in helping you establish what it is that you truly hunger for.

Think of this exercise as a big net running through the stream of your thoughts, catching all the ones that undermine you. Isn't it amazing how many negative thoughts and fantasies we engage in? What a waste of time and energy. Every time we have a negative thought and go running off with that fatalistic daydream, we reaffirm negative perceptions about ourselves, others, and the world we live in. We also miss out on this current moment, wasting it on negativity.

Becoming aware of our thoughts means that we can consciously decide if that thought is worthwhile, and if it isn't, we can shake it off once and for all. This process is like a golden retriever coming out of a lake soaking wet, noticing it is dragged down and heavy with the weight of water it doesn't need, and having a damn good shake. Those droplets of water that go flying are the old thoughts and fantasies we worry about. As we shake them off, we feel refreshed, revitalised, and aware. We are present in the moment.

It also means that we can really start to understand what it is that plays through our minds all the time, where those thoughts may have come from originally, and why we keep having them. Then we can work out what, if anything, we want to do with them.

Life is very much how we perceive it. The things we say about ourselves all the time become the truth. If all we do is put ourselves down and concentrate on the negativity in our relationships, jobs, and bodies, then we will live that truth.

A wonderful woman I know was stunningly beautiful and had legs longer than a giraffe's, but she hated her thighs. It didn't matter what anyone else told her about those lovely, long pins; she refused to believe it. She told herself and everyone else that she hated those thighs. She berated them in a highly intelligent and very funny way at every opportunity, and so this became her truth. No one could persuade her otherwise. Until she started to accept her body, remove the judgements and labels, and become aware of how often she put herself down, this could never have changed.

If you find yourself doing something similar, the thought catcher exercise would be perfect for you. Once those pesky thoughts that undermine us all have been found, we have an opportunity to untangle ourselves from them and maybe to begin to unravel some untruths about ourselves that prevent us from stepping into the now and claiming our health and happiness.

One of the best ways to do this is a technique that Russ Harris uses in *ACT with Love*. We say to ourselves, "Oh, look, there goes another thought about how fat my thighs are and how ugly I am." This one statement about what we are observing ourselves thinking about provides us with enough "rope" to detach ourselves from the thought, to decide if the thought is true or not, and then cut that rope if needed. The choice is there, waiting to be made. This becomes easier and easier with time and practice and can be applied to all areas of our life.

We all know that we learn through repetition. How many times do we have to hear something before it becomes truth? If we always hear about how smart we are or how pretty we are, then the likelihood is that we will agree and take this on as a truth. The same thing happens with our own thoughts. If we tell ourselves enough times that we have thighs dimplier than a sea sponge and that we are therefore ugly and unlovable, we will believe it. It will become truth, and all the cells in our body will go out to prove we are correct.

Labels Aren't Just about Fashion

What You'll Need

- a journal
- strips of paper
- a pen

What Next?

For the next few days, journal any everyday negative thoughts you may be having. These may be thoughts you have about people, yourself, programs you watch, or things you have done. When you are done, group them into categories and give each group a label. Now sort them into columns with the appropriate label at the top of each column. There is an example below.

Ugly Thoughts	Unlovable Thoughts	I-Hate-Pat (or whoever it is you may hate or dislike—sorry to all Pats) Thoughts	This-Is-Too-Hard Thoughts
I have the fattest thighs on the universe.	I hate it when I nag like that.	Pat is a right pain the rump.	I am too tired to do this.

My boobs are saggier than two socks with tennis balls in them.	Why won't anyone call? Well, why would they? I am so boring.	I wish she would just shut up.	I really can't do this.

These are some of the truths you have created in your life. Perhaps you have smacked labels on yourself, others, events, places, or things you have done. You have both created the label with these thoughts and justified the label with them. Each negative label is like a stick that pokes you, breaking the skin, poisoning you, and leaving behind a festering wound. If the label is about yourself, then each time you have a thought related to it, the wound festers. If the negative label is about others, every time you have a related thought, you further sabotage the opportunity to have a meaningful, constructive, loving relationship with them.

Creating Your Own Designer Labels

What You'll Need

- a pen
- paper

What Next?

Take each label and write on a clean piece of paper, "The myth I have created is that [this person] is [insert label], but what I really want or need is [insert what you really hunger for or need in the relationship]."

There are two ways to change these labels. Choose which you think would work best in the circumstances. You may even wish to do a combination of both. Labels are generally things we have had for a long time, and as such, there are patterns of behaviour and interaction associated with them. These patterns have been around for a long time too. Now, you are trying to get rid of this label and replace it, perhaps with something positive, hoping to eventually get rid of your labels altogether and just enjoy being. This can take a long time, but it is so worth it.

Option One

Create an action plan to change this label you have created for yourself. For example, if you have labelled yourself as an emotional eater, what steps can you take to reverse this? Do this for each label you have given yourself.

Option Two

Each day meditate on what it would be like to be without these labels. Just allow the images of yourself to flow through. Over time, you will start to shed these labels.

No one is the person they were five minutes ago. New thoughts and experiences happen every minute. They shape the way we think, feel, and experience our lives. So regarding ourselves the same way we did when we were teenagers, when our husbands left us, or when we were mums to little people is a waste of time. We are just who we are—just like cake is just cake. Delicious though it is, it is not love. We are not the labels we give ourselves. The thoughts, actions, and words that flow through us in these wonderful lives of ours are simply thoughts, actions, and words.

Then there are the labels we give ourselves due to the roles and jobs we have. Peel off the labels of friend, mother, daughter, colleague, or manager or bossy, controlling, fat, lazy, ugly, jolly, nagging, happy, etc. Just get rid of them and start sensing you. Really, just allow yourself to be. This is wonderfully liberating. We are not our labels. We are just that being that resides deep within. Once we stop describing ourselves in terms of labels and categories, we can be ourselves. When we identify with a role too much, then we can take on the baggage we perceive to be associated with the role.

For example, one of my clients was a very successful career woman. Then she had children and decided to do one of the toughest jobs ever: that of a stay-at-home mum. This was definitely the right thing for Tina. But what she also did was dress how she thought she should dress as a housewife. She spent her time the way she felt she should as a housewife. She spoke and acted as she felt a housewife should. She had to deal with all these associations she had about being dowdy, boring, and uninteresting to people—and a failure. So, because her heart ached with grief about her new role, even though she knew it was what she wanted to do, she ate to soothe the grief. It was only when she let go of her own perceptions that she had attached to the label of a stay-at-home mum and threw the label away altogether that she stepped into her true self. She is now thriving, as is her family.

The pose or asana below is another version of savasana. It is the corpse pose, and it explores what it is like to be without labels and just be. To reconnect with that self of yours and just hang out. You might know it as the pose done at the start or end of a yoga class, depending on the style you do. You can read through this and then get to it or download the prerecorded version from www.pathtocontentment.com.

Savasana Practice: Letting Go of Labels

Things You'll Need

- a blanket
- a yoga mat or towel
- a timer

Optional

- socks
- an eye bag

(If you have a spinal injury or a sore back, there are some modifications on the website.)

What Next?

Set the timer to ten minutes. Lie down on a mat on your back with your blanket tucked in snuggly over you. It is really important that your feet are cosy and warm. Your legs should be outstretched and your feet flopped out to the side. Let your spine and back settle into the mat softly with a gentle sigh. Extend your arms loosely from the shoulders away from the torso at a slight angle. Your palms should face upward, if that is comfortable for you. Relax your neck and rest your head lightly on the mat. Keep your eyes gently shut and your mouth open with the tongue relaxed in the back of the throat. Let your entire body settle into the earth.

Become aware of the breath—the flow of air coming into your nostrils and back out. Just focus on this for a moment, allowing all other thoughts and sensations to drift away. Then gather up your awareness and draw it down to your feet. Starting at the toes, make your way up your body with the following statements: "I bring my awareness to my feet. My feet are soft, and warm and heavy. I bring my awareness to the soft fall of my calves. My calves are soft, warm, and heavy."

Do this all the way up to your head. Then say, "I bring my awareness to my body. My body is soft, warm, and heavy—heavy into the floor, settling like a feather to the floor." Allow yourself to take a loose, languid step into that deep, deep peace, and start to surrender to the breath. See a photographic image of yourself like a paper doll. There is a large stack of these images of dolls piled up in your mind. On each breath, allow one of the paper doll images of you to go up in flames as you say to yourself, "I let go of my roles," listing all the roles you may play. Then say to yourself, "I surrender and release all the labels I give to myself." Insert any words you would use to describe yourself. Note that this does not mean that you don't have those qualities. What it means is that these qualities do not define you. Say to yourself, "I let go of all my responsibilities." Then just lie there, allowing yourself just to be. Let your awareness venture into nothingness for a while. Let yourself soak it up.

This is the true you. This is the experience of self. Learn to tune in here. This deep peace and sense of comfort and knowingness is present anytime you wish to come here.

Then, when the timer goes off, roll onto your side and rest here a moment. Slowly get up and breathe deeply.

Sometimes, our baggage is caused by not being true to ourselves—not intentionally, but because we define ourselves by how others see us rather than who we know we inherently are deep inside. I had a friend whose voice changed depending on who she was talking to. She would alter the way she said certain words to suit the person, even her body language and the way she stood. You can see this yourself with some television personalities or salespeople.

Are You More Concerned with How Others See You?

What You'll Need

- a journal
- a pen

What Next?

Grab your journal and pen and mark down each time a thought centres around how someone else sees you or regards you. Note down whether you are wondering what people are thinking about your ideas or what you have said. Notice how often, if at all, you change your behaviour, the way you talk, or even the sound of your voice to accommodate different people. Do you sugar-coat things so that you don't have to explain or talk more or because you find someone intimidating?

Often when we hunger for self-worth and love, we look for validation from others. Each tender morsel of praise or friendship is gulped down to sate our own emptiness. The first step is to become aware of it. The second is to really hone in on our own inner selves and bring them forward and into the now whenever we interact with those particular people.

So, in this part, you have begun to let go of any pain, resentment, or guilt you may be still hanging onto. This can take lots of time, so it's a great idea to come back to this section whenever things come up—not just throughout this program, but over the next few years. Hopefully, in dealing with the rot, you have become aware of the power of your own thoughts, the value you can attach to them, and their ability to create a lot of the baggage to prevent you from seeing yourself as the excellent, beautiful, intelligent creature you are. Thirdly, you have explored how your reliance on others to define who you are can influence your life and hopefully guide you back to your own inner self.

Here's a summary to remind you of the daily stuff so far.

The Food Bit

- Eat **h**eaps of veggies.

- Eat a good dose of protein at every meal.
- Add a tablespoon of oat bran or wheat bran to a meal every day.
- Limit all refined, highly processed foods, white breads, pasta, rice, and sugar.
- Eat two pieces of fruit a day.
- Have at least a litre and a half of water a day.
- Don't forget the treat every day and, if you can, make it. Fall in love with fresh delicious whole food again.
- Enjoy mindful sensory eating. Make every plate of deliciousness a dining pleasure for your senses.

The Deal-with-the-Rot Bit

- Use your journal to capture any thoughts where you berate yourself or give yourself a hard time. Usually these come before something you feel you shouldn't have done, such as eating something, not exercising, or giving up on your own pleasure.
- Begin to observe whether your thoughts and behaviours change around others and what effect their presence has.

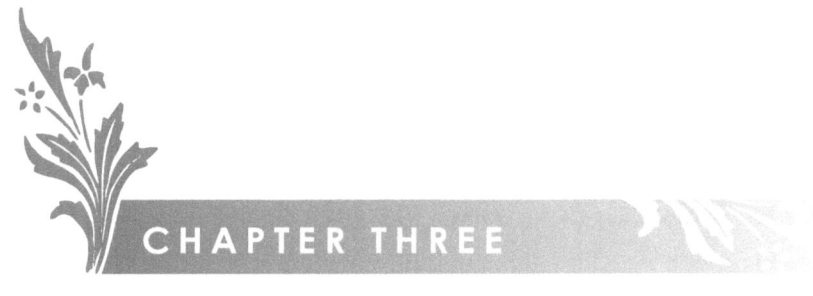

CHAPTER THREE

The Living-in-the-Now Bit

Once we start to fuel our bodies with healthy deliciousness, we begin to deal with some of the goop from our pasts that often causes us to overeat in the first place. The next step is to uncover the power of this current moment—to begin to let go of the thoughts of the past and the fantasies and fears of tomorrow and claim life now. Ideally, by the end of the book we will all be living what we truly value and believe and slurping up big, juicy mouthfuls of life as we live it.

A Quick Note

I have seen so many people give up at this stage. Self-sabotage is often a factor. I had a student called Mary. Mary was going great guns in her life. She was dealing with her emotional past, she was beginning to love herself again, she was pursuing her dreams to become a writer, and she was great at it. She looked wonderful. She glowed with happiness, and she had lost heaps of weight as a result of the above. Then she realised she was too close to success, and she gave up. She ran away for a while, stopped writing, and started the same patterns all over again. It is when success is so close that fear and self-doubt can creep up and grab you by the throat. So hang in there.

This is the time when the excuses, the justifications, and the fears may pop back up, taunt us, and nudge us to take up old patterns of behaviour. They will try to lure us into the safe world we started in. Our egos want to be right all the time. They don't like to be challenged at all. We make statements about ourselves constantly, statements we buy into and convince ourselves are correct, including,

- I am not worthy,
- I am too fat and will never be happy, and
- I am unlovable.

Those brains of ours will do everything they can to convince us that they are correct. Every time we look in the mirror or talk to a friend, it reinforces the original statement or agreement. What we are doing now is making new agreements with ourselves. These statements challenge the perceived truths that were seeded in our fears and self-doubt. It takes time to free ourselves from all that negative self-justification. Be on guard, protect what's been achieved, and allow this way of living authentically to sink into our skin and emerge as our truth. Okey-dokes. Enough. Let's begin.

Morning Meander
(This can be downloaded at www.pathtocontentment.com)

What You'll Need

- two minutes
- a good memory to remember to do it just after you wake up!

What Next?

Each morning as you lie in bed, take a deep breath. Allow the air to fill your lungs deeply. Visualise the air reaching up into your chest and emotionally softening your heart. Then visualise the air being drawn into the deep expanse of your chest cavity so that your shoulder blades slowly move apart from each other to make space for the air. Then, draw the air into your throat, asking it to soften and free your true voice with the coming day. Listen to the sounds around you—the sounds of people, nature, your household, or perhaps your neighbour's household coming to life. Tune into your body. How is it feeling? Do a mental scan of your physical limbs. How is your emotional state today as you begin the day? Breathe. Breathe. Slowly, no matter what you have to do, with great mindfulness and purpose take yourself out of bed and place your feet onto the earth. Feel yourself become grounded in the present moment, in that lovely sense of calm and stillness. Begin your day with an intention that comes from deep within. That is about being your best and embodying lots of kindness.

This scan should take but a minute and will help you enter into your body at the start of the day, rather than racing around in your head. This is an excellent way to ensure that your well-being stays a priority. When we listen to our bodies, we can then make some amendments to our day accordingly. "Oh, I am feeling a little run-down. I must take it easy today. I wonder if I can sneak in a little tea break this afternoon."

Begin each day this way.

Hint

If you are having trouble remembering to do the scan through your body and working out your emotional state before you get out of bed—because, you know, you are still half-asleep—then leave a note on the bedside table.

It may mean that you jump out of bed and then flop back in again, but pretty soon you will get into the habit.

Being in the moment is a hard thing to achieve. Our minds are so full of our inner thoughts, whirling around at a hundred miles an hour—everything from what we have to accomplish today to thoughts about others and their behaviour, from longings for the future to regrets from the past. Throughout the day, though, have you found pockets of presence where your whole being is filled with whatever it is you are doing, when there is nothing but that activity at hand? In those moments, the activity is all-consuming, and when you do it, there is no concept of time. Afterwards, there is a lovely feeling of contentedness. I love those moments.

Our minds are thought factories, producing hundreds of thousands of thoughts, most of which we happily latch onto and take for a run into various worlds—the fantasy world, the give-ourselves-a-hard-time-world, or the this-thought-must-be-truth world. These worlds are all make-believe, and meanwhile our lives are passing us by. Meditation is one of the *best* ways to help slow that thought factory down, help you reconnect with that wonderful inner self, begin to change long-standing patterns of behaviour, and help you deal with stress. It has numerous health benefits, including lowering blood pressure.

I was the antithesis of anything meditation-related. My mind was constantly on the go. I bounced around like a tennis ball on the court of Wimbledon, and my adrenals were exhausted. Now, a good few years later, I meditate for at least twenty minutes at least once a day five days a week. It has changed my life immeasurably. At first it was just a great way for me to relax. Then I began to use it as a tool to connect with my deeper self and listen to my body. Now, meditation has begun to help me really unravel some patterns of behaviour I have been trying to change. It has enabled me to be much less reactive and more open to opportunity and the moment and, most importantly, to begin to connect with a lovely deeper stillness. My thoughts are reduced considerably. I am much more aware of what that thought factory of mine churns out and which thoughts I will entertain and which I will send on their way. I also find it easier to be present with what I am doing or just with being.

So here is a section on meditation. I know time is a precious commodity, so it is broken into progressive steps so that hopefully by the end you will not even notice the time it takes you to meditate. If you really want to lose weight and claim the life you have always wanted, then meditation is as important as food and exercise.

Morning Stillness

(This can be downloaded at www.pathtocontentment.com)

What You'll Need

- a timer
- a blanket
- a candle and something to light it with

What Next?

I would recommend beginning with part A and moving to the next part each week.

Part A

Try to begin each day with a five-minute meditation as soon as you get up. Light a candle, wrap a blanket around yourself, and set a timer for five minutes. Set a dedication for your meditation for the day, perhaps repeating the intention you said to yourself as you hopped out of bed. Then, begin to count your breaths in cycles of ten, until you start to feel your thoughts slide away. Then allow the silence to replace the counting and just be. Take note of any thoughts that come in. Your mind may well wander. Thoughts about the day will come in, and you may jump onto those thoughts. That is fine. Come back to the breath. Don't judge yourself. Don't get frustrated and berate yourself. Just start again with your counting. That is all a part of meditating. Enjoy this quiet, still beginning to your day.

Part B

Five minutes of meditation is OK. Meditating for this duration will certainly help to get rid of any bad moods and help you gain that important sense of equilibrium. But to get any real, long-standing benefits, let's build up from there. (Stop rolling your eyes and recoiling in horror.) The key is to build up slowly. By the time we get to the last phase of the program, I hope you'll be seeking out that dedicated time as hungrily as I now do. This section will use five minutes of the meditation technique used in part A, and the second chunk of time will be spent on mantra. *Mantra* is a Sanskrit word meaning a phrase or word repeated to help with meditation. It has a few uses. The first is that it helps to keep the mind busy by allowing it to gently focus on repeating this phrase over and over. The second is that, if we become our thoughts and perceptions, we ought to make those thoughts and perceptions as positive as possible.

I used to concentrate really hard on a mantra, putting all my effort into repeating the phrase over and over. I have since learnt that if I allow the mantra to roll on in the background, then I can go into a much deeper state of stillness. When a thought slides in, then I just come back to the mantra, let it roll on gently, and then allow myself to go deeper and deeper. It seems to work really well.

- In this phase, the meditation creeps up to ten minutes each day.
- Pick whatever issue is the biggest thing playing on your mind. Use your journal if you are stuck and make a mantra to release yourself from it. The fewer words the better. (If I make it too long, I can never remember the thing! It drives me nuts.)
- Spend the first five minutes on breath awareness and then the next five minutes using the mantra to help focus the mind. Use your phone or an egg timer to break up the time. There is a great program called Insight Timer for anyone who has an iPhone or an Android. It has a timer that you can set intervals with as well, so you can do two minutes of one meditation and then change, for example.
- If you find yourself slipping off into stillness and not repeating the mantra, that is fine. Just let that be. There are no rights and wrongs.

Here is another option to keep things spicy; it is useful on your really, really tired days. It is a variation of the savasana exercise you did earlier.

Savasana Bliss
(This can be downloaded at www.pathtoocontentment.com)

What You'll Need

- a blanket
- a mat
- socks

What Next?

This meditation can be done lying or sitting down. Begin by just observing the breath rolling likes waves in and out of the body. As you notice the breath, notice how the mind gets snagged like a fish on a hook on thoughts and feelings. Then begin just to follow the sensation of the breath. Seek out the pause at the end of each breath. There is a tiny snippet of stillness. Linger here a moment. Allow yourself to slip into it, to lie back in it as though you are reclining back into the arms of someone you trust without question. Observe that there is no thought, no sensation—only this stillness that wraps itself around you, that settles into your very bones. Notice that as you relax completely into it, the pause grows. Allow it to fill every part of your physical being. As you witness the next wave of breath arise and the next wave of thought roll through, observe it from this expanse of stillness. As distractions come up and life begins to insist that you take notice again, there is no need to deflect these thoughts or to protect yourself—you can have stillness and thoughts at the same time. The stillness is the harbour. Anchor here today. Surrender to it.

Part C

It's time to move from ten minutes of meditation to fifteen. Hopefully, you're really starting to experience the benefits of it by now. Perhaps your mood is calmer, the awareness around everyday thoughts and responses increasing. One of the major goodies I get out of meditating is that I feel grounded and centred. I used to hate meditating. My mind was like a bag of unpopped popcorn just going into the microwave—bouncing all over the place. I thought that I was doing it all wrong and I would never "get it." Little did I realise that is perfectly fine.

With an extra five minutes, there is some more time to play with now. It all depends on how you are doing. If you are finding that you lack concentration and that your mind starts to drift off, change what sort of meditation you do every three to five minutes. Eventually you'll be able to sit for the fifteen-minute duration. Some of us, though, may have found that only one technique is required to get to that place of calm and stillness. That's great too. Whatever works. I sometimes change a few times during a session to find something that works for me. Other days I wake up and only want a meditation that focuses on the spaces between my breaths. There are no rules!

Here are some things to try.

What You'll Need

- your voice
- a pillow
- a blanket (if it is cold)
- an eye pillow (optional)
- socks (if it is cold)

What Next?

- Breathe in to a count of three, hold the breath for a count of three, exhale for a count of three, and hold the breath for a count of three. Repeat. If this is too difficult, then by all means, start with a count of two. Eventually, see if you can build up to a count of five.
- As you inhale, say, "I am inhaling." As you exhale, say to yourself, "I am exhaling." This is a great exercise I picked up from Thich Nhat Hanh.
- Or you may just want to sit in silence. These techniques are really just a footbridge to help you get to that background stillness, to stop the thoughts rolling over in the mind.

Part D

Your regular practice becomes twenty minutes now. Twenty minutes is a great length of practice and relatively easy to maintain. I hope your body and mind hanker for this brief period of calm to envelop yourself in. So far we have done the mantra, breath, and still-mind styles of meditation. For those who are visually inclined, here is a lovely technique called candle-gazing meditation.

What You'll Need

- a blanket
- an altar
- a candle and a lighter

What Next?

Sit down in a comfortable way with the candle in your line of sight. Position it so that it is easily accessible. Feel your sitting bones settle into the ground or chair beneath you, but let there be openness in your chest and heart. Do this by straightening the spine and allowing the shoulders to slide away from the ears. You may need to lean against a wall or use a chair if you have a sore back. Inhale and light a candle. Listen to the flame splutter into life. You may also detect a slightly acrid smell as you ignite the flame. Become aware of the heat that is generated from the lighter. As you move to light the candle, dedicate this meditation practice to someone you care about.

Be still. Direct the breath deeply into the body and look at the candle. Allow the candle to become the sole focus of your sight and concentration. There is nothing but the candle. Then soften your gaze a little. See the outer edges of the candle smudge. Bring your entire sensory awareness to the flickering dance of the flame. Notice if the flame is moving as if in a sinuous, slow dance or a sparky, flickering pattern. Concentrate on the colours of the flame. Perhaps there is a soft smoke wafting off the top of it. Allow your awareness to drip down to the wax pooling around the base of the candle. The soft liquid centre at the top of the candle summons you deeper and deeper within. See any drops of wax journeying down the length of the candle. Then bring your awareness back to the flame. Allow the mind to be drawn completely into the moment of now.

This blanket of stillness is present whenever you need it. Melt into the candle. Nothing exists in this present moment but you and the candle.

Emotional Reactions

Everyone has negative emotional reactions to things from time to time. Usually, as we go about our day, we do not question why we are reacting like this but just jump deeply into the puddle of the negative emotion with the intention of spitting out what we are feeling. This could be anything that doesn't make us feel safe or right. We may even find ourselves wondering why we reacted that way or wish we had more control and hadn't said what we said. Or we may feel this hollow, horrible feeling in our gut. I would often accompany it with a one-litre tub of creamy vanilla, shovelled in to soothe and comfort that dreadful feeling.

One of my clients was moodier than the ocean. Every time I saw her I almost held my breath until I saw what mood I would have to deal with that day. When it was bad, it was all about blame and raw, putrid anger, and when it was good, well, she was more effervescent than a shaken bottle of Coke. Her emotional reactions were her trap. She slathered herself in them and used her emotional reactions to things to determine how she would feel for the next few hours or even the next few days. She stumbled around like this for quite a while, unaware of the source of her unhappiness and her sense of being out of control and eating anything she wanted. Then she realised that she had a choice and could respond any way she chose in any given moment. She became conscious of her effect on others. Not only that, she began to see what came before the mood and the chippies. She began to identify her triggers.

Ever Been Called Moody?

How do your emotions affect you? Do you find you are surging around on a roller coaster of ever-changing moods? Throughout this program we have started to develop what is called the witness state of mind. Perhaps during meditation or throughout the day, you have started to observe your thoughts and to see patterns that may be leading to all sorts of behaviours and stopping you from stepping into the now and living your potential. This state of mind, where you observe what you are doing and saying, can also be used to help us maintain a sense of contentment no matter what is happening in our lives, no matter what we are feeling or what mood we are in. As Martha Beck once wrote, "You can feel peaceful even if your daughter robs a bank."

Ask yourself right now how you are feeling. Did the statement begin with "I am" or did it begin with "I am feeling"? If it began with the words "I am," then perhaps you're claiming your emotional state as a part of yourself. When I say I am angry, I am not actually the emotion anger. I am feeling anger. We are not our emotions. Our emotions are just like floating clouds across a sky. They come and go, and it is really up to us how we choose to respond when we are experiencing them.

This is much easier said than done.

Choosing the Best Response

What You'll Need

- an automated calendar system that sends you reminders (optional)
- a few days

What Next?

Every few hours over the next few days, ask yourself how you feel. This is where that calendar system might work for you. Set a reminder in your mobile or pop a Post-it note on your computer. Take a note of the feeling and the time. Try it for a week. Begin to see any patterns emerging. Also, observe the thoughts, conversations, and people who came before this emotional state or any major events of significance that occurred. Again, note any patterns. Were there any eating urges or behaviours that were uncomfortable when you felt a particular emotion?

Now, the challenge—how do we get out of a putrid funk without pretending it doesn't exist or supressing any emotions? The next step is designed to help you act in a way that honours and reflects what you value and who you truly are, no matter what your mood is.

Get Me Out of This Foul Funk!

What You'll Need

- your eyes peeled to take in any negative states
- a journal
- patience

What Next?

Take note of the negative states only. Every time you start to feel depressed, angry, grumpy, irritated, jealous, like a giant, furry-backed sloth, or just plain sad, do the following.

- Acknowledge to yourself what you are feeling.
- Step into the emotion with your breath. Allow yourself to feel it. What does grumpy feel like within you? How does it affect your thoughts, your body, and your relationships? Comfort yourself. Everyone deserves to be listened to with pure attention. Then hold yourself, love yourself, and comfort yourself.
- Identify the cause of the mood. Do this with the journal.
- Now physically release the mood in your body. This is really important. Here are some suggestions to help you physically process a particular mood.

Emotion	Yoga Poses (You can find instructions for these poses at www. pathtocontentment.com.)	Breath (Instructions are also at www. pathtocontentment. com)	Other Suggestions
Anger	Sun salutes followed by uttanasana (standing forward bend) or any forward-bending pose that brings your head lower than your heart.	Bellows breath	Jump up and down, go for a run, go outside and yell, or shake your hands up and down wildly.

Sadness	Heart-opening poses— any back bends will do. Ustrasana, or camel, works very well for me. Other options include virabhadrasana two (warrior two) and shava udarkarshanasana (supine twist with the arms outstretched).	Alternate-nostril breathing (nadi shodana) or some lovely deep breathing, focussing on the heart or wherever you can feel the weight of the sadness.	Circle your arms from the shoulders slowly, play some sad music, and just allow yourself to be with the music.

- Meditate for a few minutes until you find your centre, your home.
- If relevant, apologise to anyone you may have affected with terse words and grumblings.

Moods are tricky. Often, they attack from deep within, and many times we aren't even aware how they came to be. And they are damned difficult to change, particularly a "bad" one. But we can choose how we behave regardless of the emotions we are experiencing. As a mum, I am *constantly* practising this one. Sometimes I fail dreadfully. Sometimes that yell of impatience comes roaring out with fire and venom fuelling it. But I am slowly getting better and giving the best of me to those I love. It is really liberating once it starts to happen. I hope you find it so too.

Living in the moment means we can start to really enjoy what life is serving up to us now. We can make conscious choices that serve our higher good. We can shed our past and our future fears and fantasies and be who we really are right now.

Me? Afraid? Well, Maybe a Little

Let's begin now to work on our fears. Fears can grip us by the gizzards and literally paralyse us. I am talking about a type of fear distinct from the ones associated with our past. I am talking about the stuff that stops us from living in the now, stuff that may have come about because of something we kept telling ourselves and then started to believe. For example, there is no way in the whole universe that I would ever wear a bikini at the beach. In order to become the radiant, tantalising creature that you are, it is time to send the fears packing.

What are you afraid of? I don't just mean fears of heights or furry-legged spiders. I am also talking about those deeper fears—like being all you can be or being alone or out of control. I am talking about the fear of being disliked or without money. The subtle, everyday fears that ripple just under the skin, change the current of your thoughts, and manipulate your spoken words so much. The observations you are making with the thought-catcher exercise should start to give some real insight into those fears.

What You'll Need

- a pen
- paper

What Next?

Use the journal where you have written all the negative thoughts you observed yourself thinking in the thought-catcher exercise. Are there any patterns? Highlight key themes and common threads. Bring to mind an image of yourself as you wish to be. Allow that image to hang there in front of you. How do you feel? Then think about those common themes. What are you afraid of? What is holding you back from being all that you can be? Breathe deeply and keep asking yourself, "What am I afraid of?" Without editing it, without allowing yourself to comment on it, allow whatever comes up to come up.

When you are ready, complete the following. You may need to do this a number of times for each fear.

- If you are a visual person, then draw the fear. How does it feel inside you? What colour is it? What texture?
- If you have a passion for words, write about it. What language describes it? How does it make you feel?
- If your world is dominated by music, then make a song list or write down lyrics that express how you feel when you think about these fears.
- During each meditation session, spend a few moments visualising yourself encountering that fear and what it would be like not to have it. Over time, you will begin to change your behaviours so that you no longer fear wearing that bathing suit. Instead, you will be strutting around in it, revelling in the feeling of that sunshine on your skin.

Here is a reminder of some daily things to incorporate.

The Food Bit

- Eat heaps of veggies.
- Eat a good dose of protein at every meal.
- Add a tablespoon of oat bran or wheat bran to a meal every day.
- Limit all refined, highly processed foods, white breads, pasta, rice, and sugar.
- Eat two pieces of fruit a day.
- Have at least a litre and a half of water a day.

- Don't forget the treat every day and, if you can, make it. Fall in love with fresh, delicious whole food again.
- Enjoy mindful sensory eating. Make every plate of deliciousness a dining pleasure for your senses.

The Deal-with-the-Rot Bit

- Use your journal to capture any thoughts where you berate yourself or give yourself a hard time. Usually these come before something you feel you shouldn't have done—like eating something, not exercising, or giving up on your own pleasure.
- Begin to observe if your thoughts and behaviours change around others and what effect their presence has.
- Journal all your negative thoughts and every moment you catch yourself reaching for something you didn't really want to chow down on.

The Living-in-the-Now Bit

- Conduct a mental scan through the body and of your emotional and mental state as soon as you wake up.
- Do daily meditation starting at five minutes and building to twenty minutes.
- Monitor your moods and choose how to act when you are in a foul one.

CHAPTER FOUR

The Learning-to-Accept-and-Like-(and, OK, Love)-Myself Bit

Beginning to accept, like, and ultimately love ourselves is fundamental to having any healthy relationships, to helping you lose the weight you want to, and to living the life that you are meant to. I used to have body dysmorphia when I was a teenager and in my early twenties. I would shut my eyes in the shower so I wouldn't have to see myself as I washed. I would try to avoid mirrors at all costs. I always put others first, often at my own expense, and entered into countless codependent relationships, all because I held no regard for myself at all. Now it's a different story, and I have found I am able to give so much more to those I love, to live a much more pleasurable and fulfilling life, and to have much more empowering relationships with people because I am a bit of all right. You can too. It's OK to be tops.

Mirror, Mirror on the Wall . . .

What You'll Need

- objectivity
- a full-length mirror

What Next?

Next time you get dressed, put on those fabulous clothes, swan over to the mirror, and take a gander. There are four parts to this too. So spend perhaps a week on each part.

Part A

See yourself. I mean objectively see your two arms, your two legs, your bottom, your tummy, etc. This is yours. It is neither good nor bad. Notice what your breath is doing when you look in the mirror. Then start to deepen it. If you start to judge and criticise yourself, then just redirect yourself back to your breath. Look at yourself with curiosity and eagerness. Every morning for a week or so, practise just looking. Have a really good look. Turn from different sides and different angles. No little voices, no nothing—just look with a sense of interest.

Part B

Every day of this stage, just before you get dressed in the morning, glide on over to that mirror. This time, take the two minutes to really look at that glorious body of yours and say to yourself, "I accept my body just as it is." Try not to argue with yourself or to put a *but* in after you look at your butt. Just repeat, "I accept my body just as it is."

Maybe you are screaming at me mentally right now, "Um, hello! I do not accept my body just as it is. I want to *change* it, you bloody idiot. That's why I bought the book!" Yes, I know. But 'tis time to surrender to the way your body is right now. In this moment you have a gorgeous body, which means you can do so much. You can walk, run, laugh, make love, cuddle, and feel. Surrender and accept that body just as it in this moment. Stop fighting and struggling with those limbs and curves of yours and just accept it. Clothe it in beautiful clothes. Lather and pamper it. Care for it and acknowledge its existence with acceptance.

Part C

This is the week to begin to tell yourself all the things you like about your body. So mosey on over and have a good hard look. Start at the top and work your way down. If you struggle, think about things other than physical attractiveness. What would life be like without your arms, your thighs, or your eyes? As you say to yourself, "I like my arms," add in a *because*. We will do this in some more detail in the next exercise. Do it often enough, and you will start to reprogram any of the negative perceptions you may have held.

Part D

In this week, you move from *like* to another *l* word. No, I don't mean *loathe*. *Love*. Simply repeat the exercise from part C and substitute the word *like* with the word *love*. Be real here, and genuinely try to find a reason to love the various parts of you. The fact that you are alive is a good place to start.

The simple act of repetition and the use of a visual prompt to reinforce what we say are great, practical ways to start to reprogram any negative self-perceptions.

Making Peace with Your Body

'Tis time to make a truce with our bodies. I will go even further than that—it is time to not only step into our skin and claim it as our own, but to forgive our body and start to nourish and love it as well. Until we do this, we will not step into our authentic selves. How can we be who we truly are when we constantly deprive and punish our bodies with diets, abusing words, and self-deprecating comments?

Sometimes we wage a war on our bodies, hating them and blaming them for our lack of success, sex, love, and happiness. One of my friends is a brilliant woman. Yet she felt lacking in love and desperately unhappy. She blamed her body for the absence of a relationship in her life, so she waged a war with it, filling it with unhealthy foods, never exercising, and then berating it constantly in the mirror for how it looked. In her mind, it was all her body's fault that she felt alone and couldn't "catch herself a man." It went even further so that she was soon sleeping with men to get just some form of affection. When they failed to return her calls, she would again blame her body for the failure in the potential relationship. "It must have been because I am so fat or my thighs are saturated in cellulite," she would justify. So she would reach for a tub of caramel crunch swirl ice cream to numb her sorrows and pain.

Yet her battle was really all about her lack of self-love. She found that when she began to love and respect herself, this would attract people into her life who loved and respected her. As a by-product, when she began loving herself, she also began to eat well and exercise. Her weight and her body had absolutely nothing to do with her failure to find love. Her hate for herself, which she directed specifically at her body, had everything to do with it.

The first step for me in weight loss was to realise that it was not my body that was doing this to me. It was my thoughts! The endless beliefs and perceptions we have created about ourselves are what do it. It is not our bodies' fault. Thoughts like *I am unlovable, I am worthless,* and *I am afraid to be all I can, as no one will love me* are what does it. So we hunger. We hunger for love and stuff that hunger full of food, and in doing so, we create a safe haven behind the fat. The love we need, though, can't come from anyone but ourselves.

When we were young, we often saw our bodies as perfect. We lived in them. We didn't give our weight a second thought. They were a physical expression of who we were, and joy ran riot over our skin when we ran like whippets, skipped, and lived. Those bodies were loved. They were the physical manifestation of who we were! They were joy, light, truth, love, trust, and laughter.

It is time to finally make peace with your own body. It is time to start to see that it is not your body that you hate so much. It is time to send yourself a little kindness.

Body, I'm Sorry

(This exercise is available as a download at www.pathtocontentment.com)

What You'll Need

- a mirror where you can see *all* of you, from your twinkletoes to your tresses
- an open mind
- moisturiser (preferably one without parabens or petrochemicals)

What Next?

So, my friend, get nudey-rudey. Sidle up to a mirror and take a good, hard look. Look at yourself from the top of that delightful head to the hairs on your toes.

Breathe in deeply and slowly exhale. Where do your eyes want to focus? Do they go straight to the "bad" bits? Really tune in with loving curiosity to what your mind is saying when you look at each part of yourself. Do the stories start up again? How cruel are you to yourself? It is rare, I bet, that you would say these things about anyone else, yet for some reason it is OK to say them to yourself. You are worthy. You are beautiful, and your body is waiting for you to reclaim it, to connect again, and to be tender and loving towards it.

Note: There are two versions of this available, one for those who haven't had children and one for those who have.

Get some moisturiser, and start to massage in the cream. Start at your feet in loving circular motion. Then say to yourself or (play the download), "I love you, feet, for the roads you have taken me down." Make nice, smooth, upward strokes with the lotion. "I love you, calves and ankles, for being able to kick my heels up and have a laugh and to charge after what I truly believe in.

Continue the smooth upward strokes saying to yourself, "I love you, thighs—yes, I really do—for being able to climb over mountains and hills, both physically and spiritually, for being my strength, and for allowing me to stand tall.

Moving up to the bottom, begin to rub the lotion into your cheeks in a circular pattern. Say something like, "I love you, bottom, for your shapely curve, cheekiness, and fun and for always offering me a seat to ponder the world from.

When you come to the hips, continue the massage in a circular pattern. This time you could say something like, "I love you, delectable hips, for reminding me I am a woman, for changing shape when I carried a child (if applicable), and for helping me keep things together.

Once you come to the stomach, begin to rub the moisturiser into your skin in a circular clockwise direction. The accompanying affirming statement is, "I love you, tummy. You truly are a place of wisdom and spiritual nourishment. I love your ability to expand with child and contract again and to sustain me when all else goes wrong.

The chest is a delicate area. Massage each breast in a circular pattern towards the heart. This time you say to yourself, "I love you, breasts, for making me a woman, for the nurture you may have provided, and for the love and sensuality you have allowed me to feel and express.

Moving round to your back now, make small circles on your lower back and as much of your back as you can. The statement of self-love is, "I love you, spine and back, for giving me the strength to stand tall through my personal pain and any challenges thrown my way and for allowing me to bend over backwards at times when I didn't think I had it in me."

The massage then moves to your hands. You would say to yourself, "I love you, hands, for allowing me to caress, express, and create."

Then adopt long, smooth upward strokes on your arms and say, "I love you, arms, for the ability to cuddle, to dance, and to release my heart."

Make your way up to your shoulders. This is usually an area of a lot of tension and state, "I love you, shoulders, for carrying my baggage and what sometimes felt like the weight of the world around and for helping find my inner strength.

Once you get to your neck, use those long upward strokes again and say, "I love you, neck and throat, for giving me voice and for helping me take risks and speak up when I thought it was right to do so.

The face is a combination of massage strokes. Use upward strokes from the chin to the temple. Follow that with small circles on your temples and across your forehead and then circles from your brow bones around each eye socket. The accompanying mantras are, "I love you, face. I love the map of my life written on my skin—the lines that tell me of my laughs, my eyes that tell me who I truly am and what I am truly thinking, my cheeks that love to rise up in a smile, and my mouth that loves to kiss, savour, smirk, and laugh.

Finish up by saying, "I love you. Thank you. I love you, and I am so, so sorry for giving you such a hard time."

Our bodies are designed for us to be healthy and well. Our body hungrily seeks balance and health and vitality, and it tells us in heaps of ways when it is not getting what it needs.

Self-Love Salve

Every day, when we look in the mirror to get ready for our day, after we have just finished a meeting or had an intense conversation, when we have a shower or see someone whom we perceive to be a looker, we judge ourselves—and more often than not, we do so in a negative light.

As Marianne Williamson says in *A Course in Weight Loss*, "There is no way to surrender our weight without surrendering our subconscious belief that we're better off weighing too much."

Our innate, burning desire to shed the kilos is actually our true selves hungering for us to shed the pain and self-abuse and become more of who we truly are—to become complete. Time and time again, I have seen that what we truly hunger for, the reason we become these ravenous wildebeest, is love—self-love, love from others, just plain, old *love*.

I have gone on and on about letting go of our labels and feeding ourselves with what we truly hunger for. But now it is time to break ourselves open a little and get to the heart of the matter. It is time to acknowledge and welcome back that part of us that we hate so much—our bodies!

What You'll Need

- a pen
- paper or a journal
- an envelope
- a candle
- nice music

What Next?

It's time to write yourself a letter. So get yourself in the mood, light the candle, and put on some music that makes your hips sway. You are writing to a particular aspect of yourself: your body. "Dear me" is a good place to start. Now, before you stare at "Dear me" for the next twenty minutes and fantasise about that choccy biccy in the fridge, remember that you are writing to an aspect of yourself as though you writing to your best friend—as though you are trying to make amends with your best friend after an argument or a separation.

Think about all the horrible things you have said to yourself about your body. List them down in your letter and apologise to yourself. Explain why you said those things and offer comfort. Here is a letter I have written to myself as an example.

Dear me,

It has been such a long time since we have talked, hey? I thought it was well and truly time to put pen to paper and reach out. I have treated you so poorly. I have resented you for the cellulite on my thighs and the tummy rolls. I have hated you for my stretch marks, and I blamed you for what you did to me after my pregnancy.

Every time I looked in the mirror or met someone new, all I could think of was how ugly and unattractive I was—that this person would never "see" me, you know? He or she would never notice me, never love me—and it was all your fault. Oh, I gave you such a hard time. I stuffed you full of pizza, chips, and chocolate to make you numb. I would just shovel it in again and again.

There are so many reasons. I wanted to silence the pain. I wanted to be comforted. I wanted to feed my hunger for self-acceptance and love. I wanted to escape from what I was truly hurting from in my past. I wanted to become invisible.

So I would medicate with food and then punish myself with self-abuse afterwards at what I had done. I am so sorry. I am sorry for what I have done to you. I am sorry for not accepting and dealing with my pain. But this time I am here for you. You will be OK. You will be safe.

You really are a good egg. I am going to accept you, love you, and treat you well—I mean us.

Let's give it a shot, hey?

Love,

Zali

Your own letter may well be very different. Here are the main goals.

- List the ways in which you have abused or neglected yourself.
- Explain why.
- Offer comfort.
- Write a commitment to yourself and explain how this is different now.

Then, at the very end, say to yourself, in your own words, "I welcome all parts of me back into the whole. I am lovable, and I love myself."

Write this down on a piece of nice paper and place it in an envelope in your journal.

Now is the time to accept your body again and start claiming it as your own.

Here is a reminder of some daily things to incorporate.

The Food Bit

- Eat **h**eaps of veggies.
- Eat a good dose of protein at every meal.
- Add a tablespoon of oat bran or wheat bran to a meal every day.
- Limit all refined, highly processed foods, white breads, pasta, rice, and sugar.
- Eat two pieces of fruit a day.
- Have at least a litre and a half of water a day.
- Don't forget the treat every day and, if you can, make it. Fall in love with fresh, delicious whole food again.
- Enjoy mindful sensory eating. Make every plate of deliciousness a dining pleasure for your senses.

The Deal-with-the-Rot Bit

- Use your journal to capture any thoughts where you berate yourself or give yourself a hard time. Usually these come before something you feel you shouldn't have done—like eating something, not exercising, or giving up on your own pleasure.
- Begin to observe if your thoughts and behaviours change around others and what effect their presence has.

The Living-in-the-Now Bit

- Do a mental scan of your body and your emotional and mental state as soon as you wake up.
- Meditate daily, starting at five minutes and building to twenty minutes.
- Journal all your negative thoughts and every moment you catch yourself reaching for something you didn't really want to eat.
- Observe your moods and choose how you will respond.

The Learning-to-Accept-and-Like-(and, Okay, Love)-Myself Bit

Get used to looking at yourself in the mirror every day without judgement or criticism, and gradually add more loving observations to your self-talk every time you look in the mirror.

CHAPTER FIVE

The Exercise Bit

S ally used to *hate* exercise. No, I don't think she would even credit the term with so much emotion. She held it in this apathetic sort of regard. She associated it with all the things and all the people she was not. This really related back to her childhood. Only a "certain sort of person" was physically fit, loved sport, and was good at it. Sport and exercise were in the same dung pile in her world. That dung pile was one from which, as a child with myopic vision and lack of motor skills, she was excluded from—but one she would have dearly, really loved to step into. It comes with social acceptance—an instant group of friends and support. In the world of a child, the primal things like physical adeptness equalled superiority and popularity.

This is a prime example of the power attached to simple concepts like exercise. What do you feel when you consider the concept of exercise? What labels have been stapled to it? What emotions are attached to those labels? Some people see it as an area of failure, a reminder of how far they have fallen off the path to wellness, and recall how they used to be this super fit person, so they avoid it. Others think fitness is a world that only the elite and adept can inhabit. Others avoid it because it means entering their bodies, and right now that is just too painful.

At the end of the day, exercise is really just the movement of our body. It is an invitation to slide back into our skin and reclaim our muscles, bones, hips, and thighs. All the other stuff we attach to it is simply our stories—stories and perceptions from our past.

Here are some strategies to use to help change some of those perceptions.

Bye-Bye, Unsweet Perceptions

(This exercise is available as a download at www.pathtocontentment.com)

What You'll Need

- a few minutes
- a comfy chair

What Next?

Sitting comfortably, gently close your eyes. Visualise the word *EXERCISE* in big capital letters. Allow yourself to swill the word around in your mind. Welcome any images, experiences, words, music, and feelings that roll up. Try not to judge or analyse. Just let the imagination roam free wherever it may go. Imagine now a large pair of scissors. Those scissors are now cutting away all those old associations that have become attached to the concept of exercise. The word is now standing there by itself, clean and fresh. It is printed in crisp, black letters on stark, white parchment. Now, see an image of yourself naked, just as you are, without judgement or editing. Pop a smile on your face. Breathe normally for a few minutes. As you inhale, the word *exercise* will be breathed into your very being. Welcome it in and allow it to be at home inside you. Your eyes shine with glee, your muscles relax and release, and your breath deepens. Your body is happy. Allow yourself to sit with this image for a few moments, and when you are ready, slowly and gently open your eyes.

You can also try a mantra about exercise, depending on what old perceptions you are trying to reverse. Here is an example: "I welcome this opportunity to reclaim my body and begin to use it again for wellness."

Every time you exercise, notice how great you feel afterwards. Allow your awareness to settle on how your muscles feel and what your mood is. Really start to think about how alive, vibrant, energised, and (depending on the style of exercise) calm and focussed you feel each time. The more you can dwell on the juicy goodness of how you are feeling emotionally and physically, the sooner the perceptions will alter. You'll soon be dancing around in anticipation of getting moving again.

Yoga

OK, so I am biased, being a yoga teacher and all. But yoga is one of the best ways to obtain strength, tone, and flexibility. In this program, yoga is a really important component. Here is why.

- You don't just stretch with yoga. You build muscle mass, and let me tell you, depending on what you are doing, that heart rate can get up there. It is an all-in-one workout.
- Heart, body, and head all get a workout.
- It is suitable for all body types, and whatever weight you are at is the best weight to begin at. There are always modifications that can be done.
- You can do it even if you have certain injuries, and it may help prevent those injuries from reoccurring.
- It can be as gentle or as physically demanding as you make it, using your body as your compass.

- There are *so* many types of yoga that you will find a style and a teacher (or teachers) you love.

- Yoga helps you to listen to your body. You quickly learn where you limits are both physically and mentally as you do poses. This then extends into the everyday, when instead of shutting off from your body, you begin to tune into it.

- Yoga teaches you how to get out of the constant stream of your thoughts and into the present moment. Once you land on your rump, smack-bang in the moment, you can then choose how you want to live, eat, and love. You become alive and conscious, and you can live without the fear of past hurts returning or undealt-with pain being numbed with food.

- You begin the process of self-acceptance. Wherever you are at is perfect. If you can only get your hands on your thighs in a seated forward bend, or paschimottanasana, that is perfect. Your body is tops, and you are tops right now.

- Yoga can help you make friends with your body once again. Our bodies are so often abused and battered with our self-criticism. Not only do we shut our bodies up when they tell us stuff like "Slow down," "You are getting sick," "I don't trust that person," or "This job feels great," but then we also tell them they are fat and ugly, and blame our bodies for all our relationships failing! With yoga you can learn to regard your body as a vital, beautiful part of yourself again.

- You can connect with other yoga students, reducing the isolation that so often leads to an extra bowl of ice cream as comfort instead of a person to share laugh with.

- You feel damn good afterwards. Whether it is their energised, balanced, or content, no one can deny that you feel plain-vanilla-ice-cream-great after yoga.

- Yoga releases any long-stored tension and pain from emotionally dreadful experiences; this is one of my favourite benefits. Say, for example, that every time you see your boss you clench your jaw. This then leads to neck pain and a sore shoulder. You have this pain for years. When you finally release the muscles, you also let go of the emotion that led to it in the first place. Have you ever seen someone start to cry in a yoga class and thought, *What the?* That is usually what is happening. I have seen it happen so many times now. It is amazing. Half the time you will have no idea what the pain was, and it really doesn't matter. What matters is that you finally let it go. Emotional pain and dissatisfaction are generally the cause for weight gain, and once you get to that cause, then, well, you just don't want to overeat anymore.

- When you are exhausted beyond belief, you can still do it. Just do a restorative program instead of an active one.

Now, people tell me, "Yes, but how often and for how long?" Well, start off with one session a week, and build from there until eventually you do it at least five times a week for thirty minutes to an hour. That will hopefully mean you have a home practice going. You can use books, the Internet, or DVDs, and of course you can do classes. It takes ninety days to make a habit, so if you can stick with it, it will change your life. If you have young kids, finding a stretch of time this long can be impossible, so simply break it down into ten-minute mini sessions.

Yogic Svelte

Things You'll Need

- a yoga class
- a journal

What Next?

Part A

Begin your yoga practice with an intention to release something negative from your life, something that is holding you back. This can be anything from the way you talk to your partner to the way you think about a friend, the pain you feel when you see someone you dislike, or the fear you have when you do something new. It can be the same thing each week, or it can be something different. Before you begin your practice, take a few moments and just breathe deeply. Think about the negative thing—the way it makes you feel and whether it affects others. Then set an intention to surrender and release this negative behaviour, attitude, or pattern. Every time you go into a pose and exhale, visualise letting go. When you inhale, see the opposite happen. Breathe in healing and light. Pay extra attention when a pose is particularly difficult. This may well be where some of the emotion is stored. If it is, soften and deepen the breath as mentioned earlier. Stay a little longer in those poses.

Part B

Hopefully by now you are starting to really connect with your breath. For the next few days, begin to hold all the poses for two extra breaths. This will be easy enough in a classical style of hatha yoga, but it may be more difficult in the vinyasa or flow styles of yoga. See how you do. There is usually some holding of poses regardless of style.

The reason for holding the poses a little longer is that it will increase not only stamina, but also strength and flexibility. On a deeper level, the longer a pose is held, the better you can work at releasing those old, muscular patterns. These patterns have a psychological cause, and that will be released as you hold the pose, along with any emotion that is stored there.

It is also time to begin to play with the edge of the poses. Yoga is very much about honouring and respecting the body and knowing your physical capabilities. When you have been so disconnected from your physical form for such a long time, one of two things can occur. The first is that you think you can do what you could in your youth. The second and more common is that you are actually more tentative with yourself, warier and more reluctant to move fully into a pose.

The exhalation is the bridge to moving ever so slightly deeper into the pose. When you exhale, you will allow yourself to soften into that edge and linger there. Being able to stay with discomfort is a very important process. Quite often in our everyday lives, food is being stuffed down to numb discomfort, to stop that unease from being felt. By training ourselves to be still and present with a slight discomfort (never pain) physically, we are reprogramming ourselves to stop running from pain. Instead, we should begin to linger and observe the effects of the feeling of unease and allow ourselves to feel, accept, and learn from the discomfort.

Part C

By now, you know your yoga class pretty well. You know how the teacher talks and what she means when she lovingly says, "Go a little deeper." (My response to this one often was, "I can't go any deeper unless I become a human pretzel!") You know who is in the class and who snores at the end during meditation. You know what types of postures you like (usually the ones you can swan in and out of and do really well) and those you absolutely dread.

It is time, then, to begin to observe your breath when you get moving. In times of stress or physical discomfort, people often hold their breath, when the very thing they should be doing is releasing it.

Usually, when an asana or posture is difficult, the breath is retained, as though containing our vital life force will help us get through it. When I first started doing yoga, if there was a pose I found really hard, I would often hold my breath, shut my eyes, and pray that the thing would soon be over. As soon as I got up from the pose, my breath would explode in release and relief.

What you want to move towards whenever you're holding a difficult pose is deepening and slowing the breath. Think of the breath stroking your muscles gently—coaxing and encouraging. Every time you exhale in a pose you are letting go. You're letting go of the day you've had. You're letting go of all your expectations, roles, and responsibilities. You're releasing patterns of behaviour, memories, and emotions you have stored in your muscles.

Every time you inhale you invite in release and a fresh start. You let go of anything negative you have stored in those muscles.

Take one yoga practice this week and do it without observing the breath. Just allow the breath to be normal. Notice how you feel. Are some breaths held in certain poses? Do you breathe shallowly or deeply? Where can you feel the breath? Write it down. Then, the next day, begin your practice with an intention to let go, and surrender some fear or unwanted behaviour. Then breathe deeply and slowly during your practice. Breathe in and out through the nose. Breathe out when you fold forward, and breathe in when you come upright or stretch our arms up or come into a backbend. Basically, anytime you are opening the body and heart up, you inhale, and anytime you contract or go inward, you exhale. This phase is all about releasing—letting go.

So when the breath is released, visualise letting go of that fear or behaviour that you set your intention about at the start of your practice. Notice that when you breathe this way you hold the poses for much longer. Your practice deepens and lengthens, and hopefully a deep calm settles over you. Write down how you feel now and compare it with yesterday's practice.

This can then be applied to your daily life. Whenever you encounter stress or someone whom you try to avoid comes moseying your way, breathe. As mentioned in part B, the breath, not a chocolate bar, helps us to connect with our true self, and it serves as a reminder that this too will pass. We can choose how we deal with the latest stressor or obstacle consciously and from a place of peace.

Stage D

Pick a pose that you dislike. You know, one where you roll our eyes and grit your teeth. Now is the time to surrender the labels attached to that pose. Now is the time to begin letting go of whatever it is that you may not be confronting when you go into the pose. One of the greatest additions to our practice is to always include the poses we dislike, as they will be the most revealing, the most releasing, and the most transformational. For me, it is what I considered one time to be my arch-nemesis pose, supta prasarita paddotanasana, or the bloody-hard seated wide-legged forward bend. When I first encountered this pose, I would dread it. My teeth would clench in anticipation. I would sit and make a wide V shape with my legs and try to bring my chest to the floor with a straight back and a bend that originates from the hips. I would also pray it would all be over soon, as my inner thighs screamed murder and my breath was held in a vice until it was all over. It was only when I learnt about yoga a little more that I began to actually use the pose as a teacher and to see it as an opportunity to let go of whatever experience or emotions that I had stored there. So every time I practise, I incorporate the pose. I may never be able to lay my chest fully on the floor when I fold forward, but I have made terrific progress. Some days

I am a lot tighter than others, usually when I have some instability around my home. On others I can almost plant my lips on the ground—almost!

Whenever I go into the pose, I surrender and release. I allow myself just to be and practise acceptance of what is right now.

Here are all the benefits I have discovered for doing poses I dislike:

- It is a great reminder for me that a pose is not good or bad, it simply is a yoga position. The good and bad stuff is what my mind makes up. It is a choice. This is a great reminder for me with all things in my life.
- I can get a feel for where I am in certain areas of my life. I have discovered over time that if things are tense around money or moving, I am generally very tight in the pose. I may not even be aware that I am concerned.
- I have learnt to have confidence in what my body can do. I never would have thought when I first started that pose that I would be able to nearly kiss the ground in front of me. One day I will too! (Must clean the floor beforehand though.)
- Persistence, persistence, persistence. I often used to give up when things got too tough. So much can be achieved with a little faith and practice.
- Most importantly, I have begun to learn how to cope with difficulty consciously. I know now what I do when I want to avoid something. The physical process of sitting and being with gentle discomfort without moaning, groaning, and cursing everyone and everything has allowed me to find stillness in the moment no matter what is happening physically. This is now a practice in my emotional life too. I am able to observe the discomfort and have learnt to accept it and also to comfort myself when it arises. I used to distract myself or suffocate my discomfort with food. No longer.

- I have also gained acceptance of where I am at now. Some days I can do the pose with ease. Some days I can't. When I first started, there was no way I could even begin to fold forward, let alone open my legs wider than hip width. The pose is perfect no matter what stage I am at. Its value is in the intention behind it and the acceptance of what is in this given moment and of what my body is capable of in this place in time. Again, when I apply this to my life, it is OK that I am the size that I am now. That is perfect. I accept that. I will continue on my journey, and all else will follow.

- I have also gained an understanding of my body's limits. Doing a pose like supta prasarita podottanasana has taught me how to really tune into my body and unveiled my own limitations. I've learnt to honour and respect what my muscles are capable of and to know innately when to pull back or go a little further without harm or strain.

Here are some tips for the difficult ansanas in life that I hope will apply to the difficult moments in your life.

Get into the pose. Observe what comes before you get into it. What thoughts or emotions arise? Are there any physical responses? Once you are in the pose, just feel your body for a moment and consciously release your breath and any unnecessary muscles you may be gripping in support or protest. Allow the mind to be still or say to yourself, "I surrender. I surrender." This practice is a little like the stage before in that it gets us used to being content with things that we dislike or are uncomfortable with. On each exhalation, go a little deeper. Hold the pose just a little longer that you would like to without strain or pain. Then move out of the pose gently and do whatever your body would like to next.

Tuning In

As you are going about your day, focus on the sensations in the physical body. How does it feel to move, bend, walk, and touch? Focus on the sensations underfoot. Start to look at the body as it moves. Adopt an attitude of curiosity and nonjudgement. Invite yourself inside your skin. When we focus on our physical sensations, there is no other place to be but in this moment.

Cardio Capers

In addition to yoga, cardio is an important part of the program. Cardio is just so good for the body and mind. Aim for five cardio sessions a week. Start at five minutes if that is all you can muster, and then gradually build up to forty minutes, adding five minutes every week or two.

Part A

There is no need for expensive equipment or gym memberships. Simply step outside and walk. On those days when your heels are dragging and you would rather pick fleas off a dog, get your shoes on, give yourself five minutes, and watch your feet keep going of their own accord. Make the walk a sensory feast to chomp on. Smell the scents in the air. Feel the weather react with your skin. Feel the bounce of your feet. Allow your eyes to seek out flowers, birds, and buildings. We need this to help our blood pressure, our metabolism, and our mood! Cardio exercise is imperative in helping burn fat and has so many health benefits.

Part B

Weather is one of the greatest obstacles that I have had to overcome on my path to health through exercise. Back in the old days, if it was raining, then I simply couldn't go outside. If it was cold, then it was definitely a better idea to stay inside and snuggle. What if I got a chill? Then, of course, I am heat sensitive, so, you know, walking in the heat would just be a ridiculous idea. Then I moved to Moscow.

What I learnt in Moscow is that exercise is possible in nearly every condition—even minus twenty-five. The exception was the thirty-eight degree days—oh, and the short blizzard in winter. You see, I had no car in Moscow, and I had to get a certain three-year-old to kindergarten. We would mostly walk, and on extreme weather days and in winter, I'd take him in a cab, but then I would walk home. That is when I discovered that walking in all weather is actually pretty wonderful.

What You'll Need

- a raincoat with a hood
- waterproof mascara
- gumboots
- a hat
- sunglasses
- a winter jacket
- thermals
- gloves
- snow boots
- a sense of humour and adventure

What Next?

Walk.

If there are blizzards or high pollution, or if it is the middle of the night or you have little people to take care of, here are some ideas for alternative cardio activities.

- Put on some music and dance like there is no tomorrow.
- Go swimming. Don that bathing suit with gusto and dive-bomb in!
- Do sun salutes for half an hour! Now that will get the blood pumping.
- Jump rope with your kids.
- Put your iPod on and walk up and down stairs.
- Use a hula hoop.

Part C

You are exercising away and suddenly the inner voice starts to yell, "Enough! I am tired. My legs are aching. What time is it? I really have had enough."

Now, there is a big difference between what our body is asking of us and what our fears are asking. Fears like to try to stop every step towards what they perceive as change! The body stuff will just be feedback like "My muscles are aching." You can tell the difference because the body talk will be physical sensation. The fear stuff will be procrastination. It will come as an interpretation of body response: "Ooh, I am out of breath. I will stop." "My legs are aching from yesterday. There is no way I can exercise today." "I can't hold this pose any longer or I will collapse."

We can all consciously decide what it is our bodies are asking of us. Take a breath next time it happens and settle inside for a moment. Is it procrastination and fear talking, or is it something else? If it is just fear and procrastination, visualise what it is you are trying to achieve in your mind's eye, and then, if you feel out of breath, slow it down—but *keep going.* (If you feel light-headed, dizzy, etc., then obviously stop.) If your legs are aching from yesterday, give yourself an extra long warm-up time, and then decide if you'll continue. If you're holding downward dog and your arms are tired, then tune in and hold it for one more breath (unless they are wobbling—then come down, have a rest, and get back into the pose). Start to listen to the body rather than the fears. Fears hungrily sniff out justification for stopping. They will leap onto any little physical niggle and ride it home to victory and give-up land. Fears like to fester and fantasise. Fear will speak through excuses.

Become aware of the stories and the labels given to things. Then get rid of the stories. Push them to one side and just focus on the activity. If the negative voice starts to prattle on, just observe it and say, "Oh look, another excuse is coming."

Simply focus on the sensation of exercise. Start exploring how it feels to move your body right now. Isn't it wonderful? To be able to walk, swing our arms, or get out of a chair is such a liberating thing. Your body is responsible for this.

Part D

Hopefully, by now you'll be starting to see some real improvements in the way you feel when you do cardio. Your stamina is likely to have improved, and your breath may be flowing more easily. Perhaps you're even starting to enjoy it. A wonderful way to keep yourself motivated with cardio is to set some small goals and then reward yourself when you've achieved them. Here are some ideas to think about.

- Do a ten-kilometre walk for charity or a fun run.
- Use a pedometer. This is a simple device you can get from a sports shop, or you can even download an app to your mobile phone. Set yourself a step target, and off you go. Ten thousand steps is usually the recommended target.
- For each extra lap you swim or kilometre you walk, you get to sleep in on the weekend, have breakfast in bed, or read a book.
- Get a walking partner and set yourself team goals.
- Get an iPod and download your favourite music for when you work out.

If you've got kids to care for, then involve them in the exercise.

- Have running races in the backyard or park.
- Make an obstacle course in the lounge room.
- Have a dance-off.
- Make some hurdles in the lounge room.
- Have a jump rope competition.
- Play a ball game. Balloons are good substitutes for balls when the weather is dreadful and you need to stay inside.
- Play blind's man bluff or Marco Polo in the pool.
- Set up a running treasure hunt.
- Have a star jump competition.
- Play balloon tennis.
- Roller-skate and ice-skate.
- Bush walk.
- Get a dog.

In today's world of wireless everything and competing deadlines, it is easy to forget to actually just hang in the moment.

People are working when they are sick or outright exhausted because they simply "must." Our bodies are always giving us signals as to how they are coping physically with the demands of our lives. If not listened to, the messages may reach such a volume that they affect the nervous system, which can impact our emotional well-being. Janice often knows when she is getting sick or her body is fighting something, as she gets depressed, and yet she can't identify the root cause of the depression.

The cosy synthesis between body, spirit, feelings, and that old brain of ours can only happen once we start inhabiting our skin again. Ideally, we would like every part of us operating as one efficient, loving unit. We have wonderful bodies to claim. It is time to start to feel again with them, to let our bodies communicate with us regularly, and to listen and give them what they need and want. This is our true self talking through our very cells. To do this, we must come back into the sensory land of touch. We have started doing this with our yoga practice, some of the mirror exercises, and some of the meditation work and body work.

Here is a reminder of some daily things to incorporate.

The Food Bit

- Eat heaps of veggies.
- Eat a good dose of protein at every meal.
- Add a tablespoon of oat bran or wheat bran to a meal every day.
- Limit all refined, highly processed foods, white breads, pasta, rice, and sugar.
- Eat two pieces of fruit a day.
- Have at least a litre and a half of water a day.
- Don't forget the treat every day and, if you can, make it. Fall in love with fresh, delicious whole food again.

- Enjoy mindful sensory eating. Make every plate of deliciousness a dining pleasure for your senses.

The Deal-with-the-Rot Bit

- Use your journal to capture any thoughts where you berate yourself or give yourself a hard time. Usually, these come before something you feel you shouldn't have done—like eating something, not exercising, or giving up on your own pleasure.
- Begin to observe whether your thoughts and behaviours change around others and what effect their presence has.

The Living-in-the-Now Bit

- Do a mental scan of your body and emotional and mental state as soon as you wake up.
- Meditate daily, starting at five minutes and building to twenty minutes.
- Journal all your negative thoughts and every moment you catch yourself reaching for something you didn't really want to eat.
- Be the best you can be despite your mood.

The Learning-to-Accept-and-Like-(and, OK, Love)-Myself Bit

- Get used to looking at yourself in the mirror every day without judgement or criticism, and gradually add more loving observations to your self-talk every time you look in the mirror.

The Exercise Bit

- Incorporate yoga into your week, starting at one session a week and eventually building up to five a week for thirty minutes to an hour.
- Start to build some cardio into your day. Begin at just five minutes five times a week, and then increase that time by five minutes every week or so until you are doing five forty-minute sessions a week.

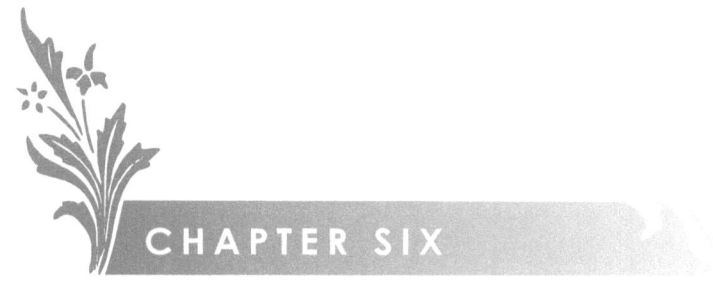

CHAPTER SIX

The Making-the-Home-a-Reflection-of-You Bit

Our physical environment is a reflection of how we see ourselves. It can also deeply influence our mood and motivations. It affects us and we affect it. This includes all environments that we inhabit: work, home, car, garden—anywhere we create or live in. From here on in, why not create an environment that honours who you are? Just as the way we act is a reflection of what we value, what we have in our physical environments and the state they are in is a reflection of who we are and what we value.

A Vision for Your Home

What You'll Need

- pictures of things you would love in your home or images of rooms you love from magazines
- pens and paints
- glue
- essential oils or incense

- music
- a journal

This exercise can also be done paperlessly on websites like Pinterest.

What Next?

Pop your music on and burn those oils. Then, room by room, write each of your physical environments that you dabble in on a separate page. Consider your home, garden, car, and workplace. Go through and create a vision for how you would like each of these to be. Slap some glue down and cut that picture out. Get creative. What would the space feel like? What would the space be used for? How would the room look? Use words, images, and styles.

The Good Stuff

What You'll Need

- your most luxurious linen
- your most fashionable cushions
- your most beautiful vases
- your best crockery, cutlery, pots, pans, knives, etc.
- your schmickest office stuff
- the prettiest smelling soaps
- your best everything!
- your favourite music
- your most precious essential oils
- those beautiful, dust-collecting candles

What Next?

Go about decking your home out with all your best stuff right now.

- Put the best linen on the beds.
- Scatter the softest, comfiest cushions around.
- Play all your favourite music.
- Fill vases with flowers from the garden.
- Get the artwork hidden on top of the cupboard down and hang it.
- Frame and hang the photos that make you burst into a grin.
- Change the lights that don't work.
- Light those candles that sit around just for decoration's sake or until someone "good" comes to visit.
- Use the best saucepans, tablecloths, placemats, cups, glasses, crockery, and cutlery.
- Get those yummy soaps saved for special occasions out and enjoy washing with them.
- Start to put out anything that's the "best," including skincare or perfume only worn for special occasions—spray it on you and in your underwear drawer.

These things are here to be used, loved, and cherished. It is our awareness when we use them that will make them so precious.

As mentioned earlier, the physical environment is often a reflection of how we perceive ourselves and how things are going in our life. If things are crazy-hazy, then generally some part of the house (or perhaps the whole thing) is in utter chaos. If you really hate your job, for example, then perhaps you will find there is lots of household administration not being done. If your soul aches from lost love or the fear of losing someone, perhaps you will find that you hang onto everything ever given to you so you can replace that love.

Seek out the places in your home that you avoid like the plague—you know, the ones you pretend aren't there or that are in the too-hard basket. These are generally places where we store all the clutter, the items that have no home, and all the memorabilia like old letters, cards, and trophies. What about the place where those rainy-day things pile up, homeless, alone, and waiting for some attention again—just like those petty issues, conflicts, and misunderstandings that are piling up? They are waiting, hanging around to be sorted out in our own mind or to be finally thrown away.

I often find that if things aren't moving in my life, when I feel they are stagnating, if I do some physical clearing of clutter and tackle the very things I am purposely ignoring, then things get moving again.

Dealing with the Dreadful

What You'll Need

- a watch
- a big roll of garbage bags
- music
- cleaning stuff
- imagination

This section draws inspiration from Peter Walsh's book It's All Too Much. *He is a guru in this field. He has a heap of excellent books, and one is focussed on the correlation between weight loss and clutter.*

What Next?

Zip around and take photos of all the cluttered, too-hard zones in the house, along with the garden, workplace, and car.

Then, one night, have a quick look through your vision for each room you did earlier. How do you feel when you see these pictures? What do you think each room and area in the house says about you? What does it say about the family or about work? Take some time now and write what you'd like each room in the house to be.

For those areas where you quickly shut your eyes and shove things in, what happens when the door is opened and you just look? Do you feel overwhelmed? "It is too hard and just plain boring" is often a thought that comes to my mind. Is it the same for you?

Take one room at a time and declutter it. Spend just fifteen minutes on each room. Set a timer so you don't go over. This takes an amazingly small amount of time, and what a difference it makes! The first thing to do is to look at the vision board or at your Pinterest boards and take a few moments to set the intention and remind yourself of what you are doing and why. Zoom around and, without too much thought, grab the garbage bags and fill them with all the rubbish. In some more bags, put any stuff that can go to charity and then finally all the stuff that could be sold. The idea is not to give it too much thought. It is a bit like quickly brushing up our appearance before going out. This is all about fun. Play some music and have a laugh.

Pop the following into the garbage bags:

- Stuff that hasn't been used in twelve months but that you simply *can't* bear to throw out in case it's needed—particularly magazines, torn-out articles, and catalogues, which continue to be my downfall.
- Anything that isn't liked anymore. So what if that vase is from Aunty Maria? A home is not a gallery that pays homage to other people's gifts.

- Things that are old and broken. That includes chipped and cracked crockery.
- Any things that have been put away and any memorabilia. Pay attention to the stuff in those boxes in the attic and garage. This includes yearbooks, school ribbons, trophies, certificates, birthday cards, mobile phone chargers, electronic accessories, dresses, and old teddies. Yes, old teddies!
- The things that haven't been used or worn for twelve months or that there are too many of—clothes and shoes, kitchen utensils, toys, books, linen, towels, tea towels, cosmetics, creams, underwear, swimsuits, jewellery, crockery, cutlery, etc. We only use one pair of scissors, one hairbrush, one set of tongs, one rolling pin, and one hairdryer at a time. You get the picture.

As soon as you are done, give it a damn good scrub physically and energetically! Wipe, dust, soap up, and vacuum. Make the space sparkle with cleanliness. Make an intention for the room and spray your favourite smells, or burn a scented candle and play some music if that suits the mood.

Now let's tackle the hoarding and stuffing places. Big breath. Try not to think about it too much. Just decide to start and get busy. Tackle these areas as though they are separate rooms. Do one area at a time and only fifteen minutes a stretch and see what happens. Dig into those cupboards, drawers, garages, spare rooms, and cars. Get your stuff organised and your to-do list pumping.

Our belongings do not define us. They do say a lot about how we see ourselves, but they don't determine who we are. It is just stuff. Physical objects are just that. But we seem to like to attach emotion to them, and they take on special meaning. That special meaning and memory will always be there; the object really is inconsequential. For example, I kept the skirt I wore on my first date with my husband for about eight years. I never wore the skirt; I just secreted it at the bottom of my drawer. Sure enough, I took it out one day and asked my husband if he remembered the skirt. "Well, um. Is that a skirt you wore when we first met or something? Why do you still have that?"

Why was I hanging onto the past with a skirt? I still have the memory. An item can be used an emotional reminder, but that doesn't mean I need to keep it.

Out with the Tatty

What You'll Need

- more garbage bags
- a timer
- anyone you can con into helping—or pay with sandwiches and homemade lemonade in exchange for their help!

What Next?

Now you are digging a little deeper and filling those garbage bags with all the tatty stuff. That means holey towels, sheets, cloths, curtains, bath mats, tea towels, doilies, tablecloths, serviettes, socks, T-shirts, jammies, shoes, bags, ironing board covers, socks, jocks, blankets, pillows—anything we may well use every day that is, well, tatty. *Tatty* is defined as chipped, holey, stained, torn, ripped, and/or drooping with age and use. Out, out, *out!*

Take twenty minutes and, room by room, get rid of all those things that have been used and worn within an inch of their lives. These things represent our everyday worn-out old selves—the bruised, battered, and much-loved of us who really need to be retired now and replaced with fresh, new, hard-working, quality stuff.

Search for bargains on the Internet if anything needs replacing, or wait for sale times. Try not to keep them as rags. We really only need about six rags in circulation at any one time, not bags full.

A Day Spa for Your Home

Now that we have lots of clear space on the shelves and surfaces and there is no more old, broken, worn-out "stuff" left, it is time to spend some loving energy cleaning, detoxing, and pampering the home, workspace, and car.

Toxins, pollutants, and dirt settle onto floors and behind furniture and mark walls. Mould grows on tiles. Fly screens get filled with dust, insect remains, and mysterious fluffy bits.

You have taken the time to create space, and now it is time to cleanse that space. It is time to get rid of not only the physical dirt and grime, but also all the energetic stuff—to open the windows and let the air, sunshine, and birdsong enter the home again.

What You'll Need

- time (no more than two hours per room)
- cleaning stuff (It would be great if you had ENJO or used environmentally safe cleaning supplies. Two experts I highly recommend are the authors of *Spotless,* Shannon Lush and Jennifer Fleming.)
- help (Cajole, bribe, con, and reward.)
- music (Make it exciting, energetic, and inspirational.)
- a ladder

- those six rags I was talking about
- hand cream, foot cream, or plain old moisturiser
- socks
- gloves

What Next?

So often, housework is seen as a *chore*. But what about if you regarded it as an act of love—an act of self-love, in that you are taking care of what you have, and an act of love for those you live with. I always think of it as creating my sanctuary. I got this one from Oprah.

Then massage a hand cream into your hands and put on your gloves. Do the same with your feet and wiggle into your socks. There is no reason why you cannot be pampering yourself while you get busy.

Set the timer for an hour at first. Walk in and say to yourself a little blessing for each room of the house—for example, "May everyone who enters this room be happy and content." Clean each exposed surface. That means

- ceilings;
- light fittings;
- air-conditioning units;
- fans;
- walls;
- skirting boards;
- pictures;
- photos;
- windows, windowsills, fly screens, curtains, and blinds;
- floors; and
- furniture (behind and underneath), rugs, cushions, and cushion covers.

Work top to bottom and make everything shine.

When you have finished a room, put some oils to burn in there and some flowers in a vase. Done.

From Functional Space to Sanctuary

What You'll Need

- your vision board
- time
- an eagle eye for a bargain

What Next?

At this point in the program, hopefully, every living area is clear, clutter-free, and sparkly clean. So it is time to bring a little beauty into your life. It is time to bring that vision you created for your sanctuary into being.

Start by organising your space. Over time, collect things that reflect that vision, and pretty soon that sanctuary will begin to emerge.

This doesn't have to be an expensive process. It can happen gradually and consistently. Every time something new is bought, get rid of something else. Welcome each new object into the home. Clean the surface before it is placed in its new home. Look at the item and really appreciate it. If you paint the walls, then think about all the happy memories this room will have as you paint.

Bring the senses alive with beautiful smells, art, textures and materials to touch, and sounds to listen to and soothe. Transform your abode into an expression of who you truly are and a place that you love deeply.

The "Alter"

Now, traditionally, altars are places associated with religion and worship. In yoga they are sacred spaces dedicated to honouring the swamis and gurus. In Catholicism the altar is the place where the congregation pays homage to Jesus and God. There is another way to think of the altar, and that is an *alter*. This where the self-altering occurs. This is a space that is special, serene, and yours, a place where you can surrender anything you wish to alter. I don't mean your fat clothes! It isn't just about surrendering, but honouring as well—a constant visual reminder of self-love and things that you honour.

Get rid of any feelings about religious hypocrisy and ickiness and get that creative head of yours into gear. Find a space that is yours. It can be inside or outside. It can be on the floor, at a desk, on a table, or on a shelf. Ideally, it would be somewhere close to where you meditate and do your journaling.

What You'll Need

- small things that you love
- a photo of people you love
- a photo of you happy (It can be one from childhood. It can be one from now. If you can't find one you like, that's OK. Maybe choose a photo or picture of a happy place.)
- a candle that smells beautiful
- your body cream
- a vase with a flower in it
- a piece of fruit that you find attractive
- your journal
- your vision board or vision book
- the letter of forgiveness to yourself
- music

What Next?

Now, put that music on, clean the space, and place the objects onto it. Make it so attractive, comforting, and inviting that its very presence makes you want to spend time there (much like people will regard your physical presence at the end of the program). This is your place of retreat, a place that is just for you, a place where you can just be. You can connect with that true part of yourself. It will serve as a daily reminder of what is truly important to you.

Here is that list of things so far to keep integrating into your day-to-day life.

The Food Bit

- Eat heaps of veggies.
- Eat a good dose of protein at every meal.
- Add a tablespoon of oat bran or wheat bran to a meal every day.
- Limit all refined, highly processed foods, white breads, pasta, rice, and sugar.
- Eat two pieces of fruit a day.
- Have at least a litre and a half of water a day.
- Don't forget the treat every day and, if you can, make it. Fall in love with fresh delicious whole food again.
- Enjoy mindful sensory eating. Make every plate of deliciousness a dining pleasure for your senses.

The Deal-with-the-Rot Bit

- Use your journal to capture any thoughts where you berate yourself or give yourself a hard time. Usually these come before something you feel you shouldn't have done—like eating something, not exercising, or giving up on your own pleasure.

- Begin to observe whether your thoughts and behaviours change around others and what effect their presence has.

The Living-in-the-Now Bit

- Do a mental scan of your body and your emotional and mental state as soon as you wake up.
- Meditate daily, starting at five minutes and building to twenty minutes.
- Journal all your negative thoughts and every moment you catch yourself reaching for something you didn't really want to eat.
- Decide how you will act when you are in a foul mood.

The Learning-to-Accept-and-Like-(and, Okay, Love)-Myself Bit

- Get used to looking at yourself in the mirror every day without judgement or criticism, and gradually add more loving observations to your self-talk every time you look in the mirror.

The Exercise Bit

- Incorporate yoga in to your week, starting at one session a week and eventually building up to five a week for thirty minutes to an hour.
- Start to build some cardio into your day. Begin at just five minutes five times a week and then increase that time by five minutes every week or so until you are doing five forty-minute sessions a week.

The Making-the-Home-a-Reflection-of-You Bit

- Every time you buy something new, get rid of something old.
- Return to your vision board regularly and update it. As you evolve, so too will your space.
- Once a season get rid of anything tatty, old, or tired.
- Try to do that deep clean every six months.

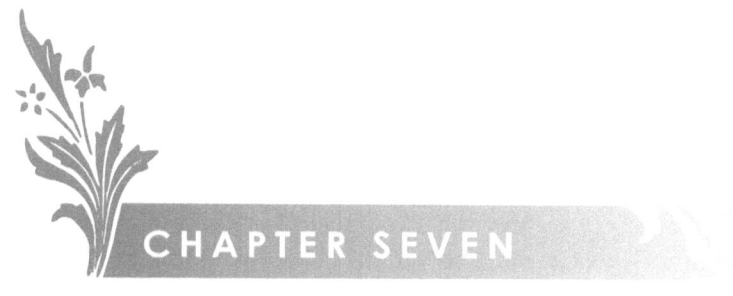

CHAPTER SEVEN

The Living-My-Life-in-All-Its-Glory Bit

This is the final stage. Hopefully by now you have inspired yourself and those around you with who you truly are. That hunger that was previously sated with cakes and chips is now being fed with what you really crave. Those labels you may have tended to staple on to define yourself as fat, lazy, and unlovable no longer apply. The clutter has been cleared from your life so that you can stride forward with clear vision and purpose, rather than be held back by the past. Your physical environment sparkles with potential. You have a regular meditation practice to harbour in daily. Hopefully you have taken proud ownership of your delectable body once again and can move it freely and with joy. Eating is now a real pleasure that nourishes, heals, and fuels you. Now is the time to celebrate, to work through some final obstacles, and to bring great scoopfuls of gratitude and joy into your life—because you are worth it.

What I Truly Hunger For

This little cherub of an exercise takes us to the heart of why we overeat. By now, after all the journaling and dealing with your rot, you will hopefully have a pretty good idea of any reasons you may have for eating jam-dribbling doughnuts to excess. Let's get to the chocolate chunk of the issue with this exercise.

What You'll Need

- if you like to write, your favourite poems, quotes, stories, and even words, pen, and paper
- if you are artsy and crafty, all those inspiring pictures, photos, and images, paint, and paper
- if you are a music person, your favourite music, pen, and paper
- if you are a touchy-feely person, your body, some music, pen, and paper

What Next?

Sit quietly and begin to meditate. Ask yourself, "What do I truly hunger for?" On your inhalation, ask yourself, "Why do I overeat and not take care of myself?" Then exhale. Continue this way for five minutes. Every time you start to think about "stuff" and notice it, just smile to yourself and bring yourself back to the question. The answer will present itself, but perhaps not in the manner you think. It may come up as a feeling, as a picture, as a quote, or as a tune or a song. So, when your timer goes off, use your materials of choice or even a combination of all of the above. Begin with your paper and write, "What do I truly hunger for?"

Then start writing, drawing, painting, moving your body, or listening to music. When you get a word or an image in your head, then put it on the paper. Maybe it's a song lyric; maybe it's a tune. For the more abstract things, replay them or read them or look at them over and over, ask yourself what they represent, and write that down. Whatever comes up comes up. There is no right or wrong answer. Take whatever comes up with reverence and curiosity.

You are calling to that deepest part of you. It may be sulking from being ignored for so long, so you may need to repeat this exercise for a number of days.

Are you surprised about what came up? If nothing came up except an image of a sugar-coated jam doughnut, just keep at it. It will happen. Knowledge is all well and good, but we will do something with it in a few exercises.

A Vision of Authenticity

It is time to rummage around and find your true calling. This is different from what you hunger for. Often what we hunger for is an unmet need, and so we feed that ache with delectable morsels and mac and cheese. This activity is about what we are meant to do in this life. This will be done in a manner that comes from the purest of intentions—in other words, with the best of hearts. It's not just about creating a vision for things that will make you purr with contentment, but it will be those things that make you want to bounce around on your bed and hug your pillow and give people a smacking huge kiss because it feels right—it feels good, and it comes from a place of kindness.

A vision board is a visual collage of what we want in our lives—our purest intentions brought into visual clarity.

What You'll Need

- magazines of all varieties
- scissors
- glue
- a blank notebook or piece of cardboard
- if you are a crafty beaver, then some other bits and pieces for texture
- music
- candles or essential oils

Or, by all means, use an electronic version as well.

What Next?

When you are ready, put on your favourite music, burn some oils or light some incense, and sit quietly. Ask yourself, "What is my calling? What am I meant to do in this life?" Allow any images to come up, any words. Just allow the mind to dream and ramble.

1. Start flicking through magazines. Have fun. Rip out any pictures you like, any words or phrases or headlines. Make a huge, chaotic, juicy pile of things you love. You can also do this with your favourite song lyrics, or, if you want to, you could make a sound collage.

2. Now begin to play and lay out your favourite images and words on the board. Get rid of any that don't feel right. This is all about your gut. Get creative. Maybe you want to go crazy and just slather pictures everywhere. Maybe you want to make a book with the precise alignment of images and words. It is all up to you.

3. Before you stick everything down, review your masterpiece. Really look hard at the pictures and make sure the board feels right. Ask

yourself, "Is this what I really want? Will it bring kindness to the world? How does looking at this make me feel?"

4. Now glue everything down, and add words and paint if you want to—whatever tickles your tummy.

5. Leave space for an image of yourself smiling and looking wonderful. Then pop one in.

6. Put the board somewhere you will see it all the time!

What I love about this is that it is just so intuitive. It is you connecting with your true self, touching base and beginning to draw that self out of the centre of yourself and into your skin.

Beautiful Me!

What You'll Need

• a good throwing arm

What Next?

Swan into your bedroom, sweep open the cupboard doors, and take out all the "fabulous" clothes—clothes that make you look great. These should be garments that fit you now, not when you were size skinny. Choose clothes that lift your emotional state up to match and reflect your true self. These are not power clothes. These are not dresses and tops that lay your breasts on a platter. These are clothes that are beautiful—everyday beautiful.

Now, if you open your doors, dig around through your drawers, and only find three things, if you can afford it then damn well dip into your savings and go and get yourself something beautiful. If times are a bit lean, try to avoid putting anything on a credit card. It won't be necessary to spend hundreds of dollars. There are heaps of alternative options, including,

- going to charity shops,
- trading clothes with friends,
- shopping at cheaper shops (The big chain stores have great stuff!), and
- making an agreement with yourself to save just five dollars a week for new clothes.

Yes, the clothes you are wearing will be temporary, but why should you look like a saggy ball of woof when you deserve to look beautiful right now? You do not have to spend a fortune. Just start with one thing. This goes for everything from underwear to pyjamas.

Let me talk about bras for a bit. If your undies and bras have holes in them or have gone from white to grey, then get rid of them. Out, out, out. If your bras do little more than cover your breasts in two sacks of sadness, then out, out, out! Go and get yourself properly fitted. It doesn't cost anything. Or check out an underwear website that teaches how to measure yourself for the right size. Wash and wear the same nice bra until you can afford to buy more.

Getting Rid of Vampires and Enablers

As you start to claim your authentic self, you may notice that some people aren't coping too well with the change. Perhaps they are used to you acting, looking, and being a certain way. This is what they are comfortable with. This is how they have labelled and stamped you. Just like a cow, you have been branded a particular way, but now you have changed herds! In fact, you have created your own breed: *you*. Sometimes, people have great difficulty when those they know, love, or work with change. They may feel threatened or vulnerable because what made sense about you and your place in their world now doesn't. They are unsure of your relationship with them or what is happening.

This is often in the case in a relationship where two people both hungered for something and shared a plate of chippies or fries with gravy to sate it and each other. It was an affirmation that it was OK to continue this way. Now, one is ready to sate the hunger, and the other is not. Perhaps they both enabled each other to eat a little more or complained about the same things all the time. This was the great thing that they had in common. If this is the case for you as well and you feel the relationship is changing, then have a chat with that friend or relative. Explain the journey you're on and how you're doing. See if they want to come on the journey too. Hopefully, they will be your biggest supporters, and you will be an inspiration for them as well.

If on the off chance they ridicule you or undermine you, try not to get defensive or hurt. This is a big change for them too. You are becoming your potential. This can be very threatening for people. If you can, give yourself some distance from them for a while. Surround yourself with people who uplift you, who support you, and who are going through similar journeys themselves. This is really important. Who we surround ourselves with is a reflection of who we are and what we value.

There are some relationships, too, that are a little vampirish in nature—when one person gives and gives and gives and the other takes. If this is the case for one of your relationships, again, reconsider the relationship, and maybe do some boundary work. It is really important at the moment that you give to yourself. You deserve it. Drink deeply from the self-love you are starting to develop and nourish your own life rather than everyone else's.

A Letter of Encouragement

With all the wonderful change being undertaken, sometimes there can be setbacks, struggles, and pitfalls. The old self-sabotage can kick into full gear. So, if that occasion should arise, it is time to write a letter to yourself.

What You'll Need

- a pen
- paper

What Next?

Take some time now. Light your candle and sit quietly. Then set an intention related to writing yourself a letter of encouragement. Allow the breath to flow evenly and smoothly, and when you are ready, pick up the journal and pen and begin to write. Write about what you want to achieve and why. Acknowledge the pain of the journey so far. Be honest about your feelings towards what lies ahead and behind you, and pour out words of compassion and encouragement for yourself.

Then mindfully set down the pen. Shut the journal and sit again for a moment. You can come back to this letter anytime you are struggling, anytime the feelings and insecurities pile up again in the coming days, months, and years.

Mentor Me Up

What about also finding yourself someone who can be a living inspiration to you? I have heaps of these people in my life. There was one woman at my son's kindergarten who always cared for her appearance and took time to look after herself. Without her ever knowing, she became a living inspiration for me to remember to care for myself too and take a little time in my busy mummy life to look after myself and put on clothes that look and feel great. Like a picture on the fridge, the constant reminder provided by her very presence was a terrific motivation.

Why not take it even further and use this exercise as a spiritual learning opportunity as well? A great source for this is someone you may have resented or envied or who may have annoyed you with their health, goodness, and fitness. These are the very people who we should embrace as a shining light of example rather than a source of jealousy. It is our perceptions of people that become our truths. What happens when, instead of putting that person down and resenting them, we instead study them with love and adopt some of the very things we are envious of?

Then there are real mentors whom you have a relationship with. Perhaps there is someone who has undergone this journey whom you can meet with on a regular basis. This could be a yoga teacher, a spiritual leader, an old boss, or a friend who loves you unconditionally. People are so rapt when you ask them to be your mentor. It doesn't have to be someone you know. You can approach an author, a leader in your community, or someone at your work you have heard is amazing. People are often so willing to act as a sounding board, to encourage you, and to share their experiences with you.

Surround yourself with people who inspire you. Trust me. You are inspirational at the moment too, and they will love to be around you.

The River

I call this one the river because on one side of the river, you will note what is important to you and how you really want to live every day. Then, on the other bank, you'll explore how you are actually living and what you really spend your time on. Then you'll launch a boat into that river and start building a bridge between the two. We spend so much of our time not living what we believe is important and instead just ticking same the to-do boxes we have always ticked.

What You'll Need

- a pen
- a journal

What Next?

Take a wee second now to write down in your journal all the things you believe about yourself and what you believe is important to you. It can be anything.

- What are the things that matter most to you?
- What do you believe in?

Don't edit or judge or question. Just get it all out. Now for the juicy bit— consider the last few days and write down the answers to these questions.

- How have you been acting towards others?
- What mood have you been in?
- What happened when things went wrong or didn't go as you thought they would?
- How did you spend your time during the last few weekdays and the last few weekends?
- How did you eat? Were you rushed? Watching TV? By yourself?
- How did you take care of yourself? Did you take any you time? Did you rest? Do you pay yourself a compliment or comfort yourself when you were upset?

Now, compare what you wrote down that you value and find important to what you have spent the last few days doing. Are there any gaps? If you are anything like I was, there are some rather huge, gaping, jagged holes.

What we truly believe and value is often different from what we want to believe and value. This is a chunky and acrid pill to swallow. How we act and what we spend our time on shows what we are truly valuing right now. What we think we value and believe is, in reality, the wish list.

Take some time now and reflect on that list of things you value. Is there anything you would add? The next exercise then makes this actionable in your everyday life.

The "I Truly Hunger For . . ." Action Plans

What You'll Need

- a list of things you truly value and want to spend time on
- a vision board
- an action plan you did earlier to address what you truly hunger for

What Next?

Look at the action plan you wrote to address what you really ache for when you overeat—the thing or things that prevented you from claiming all you could be and all that you are. Now study the vision board that you made. This was the vision that inspired you as to what your life could be if you chose. Finally, with the plan and the vision board in the back of your mind, explore what you really value versus what you spend your time on. Begin to make some real changes to how you spend your time. This is such a great exercise. It is the hands-on, down-and-dirty way to start living what you value, not just having it as a blurred, vague idea or an unwritten set of changeable bullet points in your head. This is a chance to ensure that you are living your values and devoting time to things you hold dear and people you love and adore. You are doing this in line with the vision and purpose you now have for your life and ensuring that it continues to address what you truly hunger for.

Make a number of plans if you need to. Each plan should take you one step closer to who you truly are and how you want to live this glorious life of yours. Each plan should also be about something you truly value.

After you make each plan, take the first step of that plan straight away, without even thinking about it.

This was Julia's story.

When I first did this exercise, combined with the River, I realised that I spent most of my time doing routine activities that just ate up my day. They weren't special to me and hardly added any value to my life, yet I felt duty-bound to do them. Some were even redundant things I really no longer needed to carry out. So I reworked everything. I added in my meditation time. I scheduled in exercise every day. I did this by doing my stretching and strength work in front of the television some days. I made sure that every time I washed my hands I put on hand cream. Instead of eating cakes and treaties at play group, I would bring fruit and nuts or healthy, whole-food treats I had made myself. When I do my housework, I think about the wonderful sanctuary and home I am creating for myself and my family. It then becomes a joy. When I feed my pets I take a moment to really connect with them rather than just doing it automatically. This is how I began to enrich my life and live out what matters. I still work on this every day and find new ways to do the things that matter to me and to live what I value.

Passionate Pastime

Are there things you used to love to do but now never get around to? Or perhaps you have made a list of hobbies and things you want to do, but again it sits on the fridge? As the two previous exercises have highlighted, how we spend our time is really up to us. Each decision, when possible, should be one that enriches our lives, supporting and nurturing who we are, so that, ultimately, we can give back and enrich the lives of others. When I quit the corporate world with the arrival of my wriggly, pink, Yoda-looking newborn, I soon realised that I had no hobbies except for yoga in my life. My time prior to the arrival of my son was spent mostly on food, work, television, and some yoga. When work was no longer the centre of my universe and I was in a full-time caring role for my little man, I became desperately exhausted. I was exhausted because I poured the very essence of my being into caring for my baby. The energy that I would devote to my relationship with my husband, friends, and relatives was all poured into Mr Chops. Every activity was about him. I became empty and literally ragged. It was not until I introduced balance into my life, began nurturing myself and my relationships, and added some additional hobbies into my day that I became whole again. When I started to incorporate some things I love doing into my day, my true self did a little jig, and my parenting, my relationship with my husband, and myself improved 1,000 per cent. Now, I am a busy beaver, gardening, cooking, knitting, going to book clubs, and doing charity work in addition to being a mum, a writer, and a yoga teacher. Life is great!

If we do not pursue our own passions, we miss opportunities to grow, connect, and relax. Why not take the time to prioritise you and really celebrate and live this new phase in your life by exploring what is calling?

What You'll Need

- a hobby or activity you have always wanted to do but never got around to

If you are stuck, think about the things you did when you were a kid or in college.

What Next?

- Write down all the obstacles, excuses, reasons, and justifications you have for not doing it, and then make a plan to fit the hobby in, to buy the materials, etc.
- Make that phone call or write that email to find out more about that hobby or interest and book in a class or course. You will feel great once you have.
- Don't let yourself chicken out. I am a big one for this. I make the plan, and then, when the time actually comes to do it, I self-sabotage. You do deserve to do something you love.

Giving Back

In almost all religions and secular traditions there are strong teachings on community service and charity. Giving is one of the most personally rewarding, trust-building, and loving things we can do for ourselves and for others, especially when we give when no one else knows and with no expectation of anything in return—just because we can. The act of giving is truly healing in helping to restore a sense of self-worth and in helping us trust in the goodness of life and love. It can also untangle us from feelings of loneliness. It makes us feel like we're part of something bigger. We can make a positive difference. Lives are super-duper busy, but again, it comes down to what is important in our lives and how we can show gratitude for what we have.

I cannot communicate enough the joy and contentment we can obtain from giving, sharing, and being present. These feelings multiply by ten when we help someone. What we give out will give us so much more than the recipient. There are so many small ways we can make a difference. Why not give it a go and see what happens?

Here are some ideas to spark you off. Donate some money; one or two dollars is all it takes. I remember reading in one of Suze Oreman's books that whenever she felt like she was running out of money and started to worry, she would donate some money. It sounds contradictory, doesn't it? But I now do this all the time, and it removes any feelings of scarcity or that horrible clutch of fear in my belly. It reminded me that there are those so much worse off than I am and that I always have money to give.

Maybe look up volunteering and find something that suits your time commitments, talents, and interests. Simply type *volunteering* into Google. There are whole organisations established to help place volunteers with groups and charities that suit them.

Get a group of people together to knit jumpers or scarves for shelters, work in a soup kitchen, visit elderly people, become a mentor to a homeless youth, or make cakes for neighbours going through hard times. It doesn't matter what it is as long as it is something that expresses our talents and that we enjoy doing. There is so much need out there.

One of the best places to start is right at home in the immediate neighbourhood. If the neighbours get sick, why not take them some bread or some soup? Leave them some home-grown vegetables on the doorstep. Maybe write an anonymous card to someone you know who is down. Perhaps the next time you pick yourself some flowers leave some on the neighbour's doorstep. Maybe there is a homeless person you walk past on the way to work each day. Well, this time, why not bend down, smile at them, and drop a few coins? What about making an extra sandwich and popping that into their collection bowl each day? If you have a lot of spare change, perhaps carry it with you in little plastic bags and pop them in a homeless person's cup while looking them in the eye. It's all about connection.

The Benefits of the Bristly Brush

This final phase is all about uplifting, celebrating, and pampering. So we are onto the pampering bit. One of the loveliest things we can do for our bodies each day before we hop into the bath or shower is to use a body brush. These can be bought from chemists, supermarkets, and health food stores. They're good for toning arms too.

Here are some of the many benefits of a body brush.

- It reduces the appearance of cellulite.
- It helps to optimise the lymphatic system.
- It removes scaly, dead skin bits.
- It improves microcirculation, which will help to prevent vein problems and also get the blood to all the tiny extremities of the body.
- It stimulates the hormone—and oil-producing glands.
- It helps to keep the skin nice and firm (and may assist in removing the saggy, baggy bits).
- It can help the nervous system.
- It assists digestion, as the circular motion over the belly is a gentle massage to our organs.

And I always feel alive after I've done it!

What You'll Need

- a body brush

What Next?

Body brushing is done before the shower or bath. Sweep the brush up the legs from the tops of the feet to the tops of the thighs in nice, long strokes. Then move the brush in a circular motion over the rump. Move the brush from the base of the thigh to the top of the bottom in short strokes. Glide the brush in long, catlike strokes over the fingers and up the arms to the tops of the shoulders. Tackle the torso now. Gently move the brush in a clockwise motion on the tummy and over each breast. Softer than a child's breath, move the brush down the neck and across the tops of the shoulders.

Start off gently and for a short duration, and build up to harder strokes and for a longer time.

Conclusion

So this is it. You have arrived. Look at all you have achieved. You have claimed your life again, stepped into the now with a grin, and plopped a juicy fat kiss on it. Welcome home to your body and your life! May you go on to the greatness you are destined for. May all those who have anything to do with you be blessed by your very presence and kindness. Go get 'em, tiger!

Here is a reminder of some daily things to incorporate.

The Food Bit

- Eat **h**eaps of veggies.

- Eat a good dose of protein at every meal.
- Add a tablespoon of oat bran or wheat bran to a meal every day.
- Limit all refined, highly processed foods, white breads, pasta, rice, and sugar.
- Eat two pieces of fruit a day.
- Have at least a litre and a half of water a day.
- Don't forget the treat every day and, if you can, make it. Fall in love with fresh, delicious whole food again.
- Enjoy mindful sensory eating. Make every plate of deliciousness a dining pleasure for your senses.

The Deal-with-the-Rot Bit

- Use your journal to capture any thoughts where you berate yourself or give yourself a hard time. Usually these come before something you feel you shouldn't have done—like eating something, not exercising, or giving up on your own pleasure.
- Begin to observe whether your thoughts and behaviours change around others and what effect their presence has.

The Living-in-the-Now Bit

- Do a mental scan of your body and your emotional and mental state as soon as you wake up.
- Meditate daily, starting at five minutes and building to twenty minutes.
- Journal your negative thoughts and every moment you catch yourself reaching for something you didn't really want to eat.
- Choose how you will interact with the world, whatever your mood.

The Learning-to-Accept-and-Like-(and, OK, Love)-Myself Bit

- Get used to looking at yourself in the mirror every day without judgement or criticism, and gradually add more loving observations to your self-talk every time you look in the mirror.

The Exercise Bit

- Incorporate yoga in to your week, starting at one session a week and eventually building up to five a week for thirty minutes to an hour.
- Start to build some cardio into your day. Begin at just five minutes five times a week, and then increase that time by five minutes every week or so until you are doing five forty-minute sessions a week.

The Making-the-Home-a-Reflection-of-You Bit

- Every time you buy something new, get rid of something old.
- Return to your vision board regularly and update it. As you evolve, so too will your space.
- Once a season, get rid of anything tatty, old, or tired.
- Try to do that deep clean every six months.

CHAPTER EIGHT

If You Hit the Wall—Oh, All Right, If You Just Jump off the Wall

This is a chapter devoted to anyone who may be about to give up or maybe has already. Losing weight this way is just so plain bloody hard. There, I have said it. It is hard to deal with the causes of the weight gain. It is difficult to begin to start liking and loving ourselves again and then to start to follow our dreams. This is the recipe, though, that will transform not only our bodies, but also our hearts and our lives.

It is time to revisit the reasons for losing weight to begin with. Get out that vision board and look long and hard at it. If you have completed the letter to yourself, bring it out and read it. How do you feel?

There is an exercise I adore. This one really changed my life.

What You'll Need

- a pen
- paper

What Next?

Jot down how you would normally spend your average weekday, from the moment you get up to the time your head makes a dent in the pillow. Then start to explore on paper how you would love to spend your day. What attitude would you have? What you would do?

For example, I would begin my day with a slow, luxurious stretch after my three-year-old bounds out of bed, ready to play. Then I would tune into my body and take note of how it feels physically. I would check in with myself spiritually and emotionally as well. Then, with deliberateness and intention, I would begin my day. First, I'd get the household ready for breakfast, making a blessing for each member of family as I prepare the plates and bowls and food. Then I would take some time to meditate, to dedicate this day to what is important, and to realign myself.

You get the drift.

Once that is complete, compare the gaps between how your average day is and how you would like it to be. Is there a difference? If so, why? Why aren't you living the day in the way you would like? Hopefully, most of the things would be minor, but some may be major.

Recommit to yourself that you are valuable and lovable. Is there any guilt still lurking? If so, get that old suitcase out, pack it up, and send it off to Siberia. Change is one of the most difficult things to do. Real behavioural, spiritual change is tough work but so rewarding. That old ego hates change, particularly when it leaves us vulnerable. So dust yourself off, have a big breath, and recommit—to yourself.

I read once that it is only when we are ready that we get our next lesson. So, for you this is obviously the time to deal with what is really weighing you down. Let yourself rise up and fill that skin of yours with your talents and gifts. Make it glow.

I am the ultimate procrastinator. In fact, I enjoy the anticipation of doing a task so much that I will often put it off just to enjoy the anticipation. I also like to feel in control at all times and to hide behind slothfulness in case I get hurt. So, I have been there. In fact, I visit this place regularly. It can come in many guises—laziness, boredom, other obligations, sickness, or the "just can't be bothered" excuse.

The worst bit is that we know deep into the marrow of our bones what is good for us. That makes it so much more frustrating when we do a backflip into sloth's waiting arms. What makes it even more depressing is that it is usually when we are halfway through something and about to make real progress that sloth will try to prevent us from finding joy.

I use the motto "I will just do the best I can each day." Sometimes I am too tired to pick up the teacup, so I commit to myself that I will be as effective as I am able when I am exhausted. I am now happy with that. It took awhile to surrender to what I was capable of instead of being driven by my own expectations. When I feel energised, as though I could take on the whole of Timbuktu, then I do my utmost for that day. It is not the outcome that counts, but the intention and the effort. As long as I know I did my best for this moment, that is enough.

So just do your best, taking into account how you feel in that moment, and you will become all you were meant to become.

SOURCES

Harris, Ross. *Act with Love: Stop Struggling, Reconcile Differences and Strengthen Your Relationship with Acceptance and Commitment.* California: New Harbinger Publications, 2009.

Mann, Traci, quoted by Alok Jha. "Diets don't work in the long term, says survey," *The Guardian*, April 10, 2007, http://www.guardian.co.uk/science/2007/apr/10/medicineandhealth.psychology.

Walsh, Peter. *It's All Too Much: Living a Rich Life with Less Stuff.* New York: Free Press, 2007.

Williamson, Marianne. *A Course in Weightloss: 21 Spiritual Lessons for Transforming Your Weight Forever.* Sydney: Hay House, 2010.

www.ingramcontent.com/pod-product-compliance
Lightning Source LLC
Chambersburg PA
CBHW051419280526
45785CB00003B/1082